How to Succeed at Medical School

An essential guide to learning

Dedication

To Geert and Jerry, for their support and patience, without which this book would never have been written.

How to Succeed at Medical School

An essential guide to learning

SECOND EDITION

Dason Evans MBBS, MHPE, FHEA
Senior Lecturer in Medical Education
Head of Clinical Skills
Barts and the London School of Medicine and Dentistry
Queen Mary, University of London,
London, UK

Jo Brown EdD, MSc, BSc (Hons), PgCAP, SFHEA
Reader in Medical Education
Head of Clinical Communication
Academic Director of the Student Experience
Centre for Clinical Education
St George's, University of London
London, UK

BMJ|Books   **WILEY** Blackwell

This edition first published 2015 © 2015, by John Wiley & Sons Ltd.
First edition © 2009 by Blackwell Publishing Ltd

BMJ Books is an imprint of BMJ Publishing Group Limited, used under licence by John Wiley & Sons.

Registered Office
John Wiley & Sons Ltd, The Atrium, Southern Gate, Chichester, West Sussex, PO19 8SQ, UK

Editorial Offices
350 Main Street, Malden, MA 02148-5020, USA
9600 Garsington Road, Oxford, OX4 2DQ, UK
The Atrium, Southern Gate, Chichester, West Sussex, PO19 8SQ, UK

For details of our global editorial offices, for customer services, and for information about how to apply
for permission to reuse the copyright material in this book please see our website at
www.wiley.com/wiley-blackwell.

The right of Dason Evans and Jo Brown to be identified as the authors of this work has been asserted in
accordance with the UK Copyright, Designs and Patents Act 1988.

Library of Congress Cataloging-in-Publication Data

Evans, Dason, author.
  How to succeed at medical school : an essential guide to learning / Dason Evans, Jo Brown. – Second
edition.
      p. ; cm.
  Includes bibliographical references and index.
  ISBN 978-1-118-70341-0 (pbk.)
  I. Brown, Jo, 1957-, author. II. Title.
  [DNLM: 1.   Education, Medical–methods. 2.   Learning.   W 18]
  R737
  610.71′1–dc23
                              2014049428

A catalogue record for this book is available from the British Library.

Typeset in 9.5/12pt MinionPro by SPi Global, Chennai, India
Printed and bound in Malaysia by Vivar Printing Sdn Bhd

1   2015

Contents

WITHDRAWN

vi **Contents**

About the authors

Dason Evans and Jo Brown have worked together on and off since 2000, initially at Bart's and the London School of Medicine and Dentistry where they were awarded the Drapers Prize 'in recognition of the exemplary practice and innovation for enhancing the quality of learning and teaching', and subsequently at St George's, University of London, where they were appointed joint Chief Examiners for OSCEs. They have an international reputation for their work supporting students in academic difficulty and this expertise brings insights to this book, which will benefit all students. They are recognised for their student-centred approach to learning and their passionate advocacy for the need to empower students to make the best use of the learning opportunities open to them.

Dr Dason Evans is a Senior Lecturer in Medical Education and Head of Clinical Skills at Bart's and the London School of Medicine and Dentistry, Queen Mary, University of London. He is following a career in medical education and works clinically in sexual health. He has been working formally in medical education since 1999 and teaching and supporting students since 1995. Dr Evans has strong interests in clinical skills learning, teaching and assessment and learning within the clinical environment. Through his fellowship of the Higher Education Academy (HEA), and active contribution to the Association for the Study of Medical Education (ASME), the Association for Medical Education in Europe (AMEE) and external examining duties, he has a clear understanding of the current culture in health professional education. His research interests include clinical skills, preparation for practice, students in academic difficulty and education around sexual health. He has also co-authored a book on learning in the clinical environment and, with Jo Brown, a book chapter on academic support.

Dr Jo Brown is Reader in Medical Education and Head of Clinical Communication at St George's, University of London as well as being Academic Director of the Student Experience. She began her career in nursing and management and has been teaching since 1992. She has specialised in Clinical Communication since 1998 and her passion for the subject is infectious. In 2012, she won a prestigious National Teaching Fellowship award from the Higher Education Academy. She has a particular interest in providing academic support for students who struggle or fail while at medical school. She is a curriculum designer, examiner and an external examiner, and has spent 2 years visiting medical schools in The Netherlands and Canada to explore different conceptualisations of medical education. She is an experienced mentor of teachers in higher education and runs courses on teaching and learning techniques. She has developed and delivers postgraduate courses for senior doctors on the use of advanced clinical communication in everyday clinical practice. She is a member of the Association for the Study of Medical Education and is a Senior Fellow of the Higher Education Academy. Her research interests centre on the movement of learning from classroom to clinical environment and the challenges to learning in the clinical workplace.

Foreword to the first edition

Throughout the working career of a doctor, keeping up to date is a major factor in providing good care to patients. This book aims to help undergraduates learn some of the huge number of different skills required to distil new facts and new knowledge in order to keep ahead with their learning for the rest of their professional life. It is a most unusual book in that it is written to help students develop their own skills and awareness around learning. It does not contain factual knowledge but is about the skills required to cope with medical school. It covers aspects of learning such as cognitive skills, motivation, self-regulation of study skills and the actual 'concept' of learning rather than the content for knowledge. It helps aid students to learn effectively and efficiently and even tells you how you will know when you know enough!

It does this in sections about knowledge, learning clinical and communication skills, learning how to work in a small group and, lastly, it even gives helpful advice on 'examination technique'! There are helpful suggestions about reflecting on the type of learner the student is and how to revise for examinations. Above all, it discusses the broader issues about 'living' and how to achieve a good life–work balance. It also helps with the aspirations of students and guides them to think about the future and the type of career they might like.

Although the authors say that they have written this book for students about to embark on a medical course and younger medical students, this book would also help those involved in 'teaching' health-care professionals. It certainly would have saved me a lot of time learning how to get through a medical course.

The authors both have a vast experience in this area and much of their book has been gleaned from first-hand experience. I certainly enjoyed reading it and would recommend it to all students and teachers.

Parveen Kumar
Professor of Medicine and Education,
Bart's and the London School of Medicine and Dentistry,
Queen Mary College,
University of London

Introduction

Who is this book for?

You may be reading this book because you are thinking of joining a medical course or because you are in the first few years of training. In this case, you will find this book particularly useful in helping you manage the transition to new ways of learning. Moreover, this book will be of interest to more senior students and may be of interest and relevance to students of other health professions and academics involved in their learning.

What is this book for?

Learning how to learn effectively and efficiently

During your years at medical school you will buy plenty of books. Almost all these books will cover *what* you need to know. This book is different, it concentrates on *how to learn effectively and efficiently* while at medical school and beyond. There is good evidence that helping students develop their awareness of how to learn and helping them develop a variety of learning techniques results in large improvements in performance.

Medical school is different

The learning environment at medical school is fundamentally different to secondary school or other university courses. You are expected to learn a huge amount of diverse information, ranging from Anatomy to Ethics, to become proficient in many new skills, ranging from taking blood to breaking bad news, and to be able to integrate skills with knowledge in order to work with a patient to make a diagnosis and management plan. You are expected to learn much of this without being specifically taught it. You are expected to be able to find out what you need to know and to learn it to an appropriate level, often with little support.

How to Succeed at Medical School: An Essential Guide to Learning, Second Edition. Dason Evans and Jo Brown.
© 2015 John Wiley & Sons, Ltd. Published 2015 by John Wiley & Sons, Ltd.

How will this book help you?

This book works on two levels. On the first level, it offers advice on how to learn most efficiently (study skills). This is divided up into four sections: *Learning Knowledge, Learning Clinical and Communication Skills, Working in a Group* and *Exam Technique*. On the second level, it aims to get you thinking about how you learn and when it might be best to use which study skills. This is embedded within these four sections and covered in more depth in four other sections: *What Kind of Learner Are You?, Life-Work Balance, Revision and Thinking Ahead*. By reading and working through this book you will gain not only a wider range of study skills, but also an awareness of when to use them in your learning.

What is in it?

An overview of the sections

The book starts with a chapter called *What Kind of Learner are You?*, which introduces a simple overview of learning style, helps you to think about what your preferred learning style is and how this might influence your learning. For example, you may be a perfectionist, wanting to understand the deepest nuances of everything that you learn – if this is the case, you may have trouble knowing at which point what you have learned is good enough and when to move on to the next thing to learn. By contrast, you might be a crammer, great at filling your head with facts for a few weeks before your exams, ready to forget shortly after – if this is the case, the volume of study may well overwhelm you, however good your short-term memory.

The chapter on *Learning Knowledge* covers how to make the most of lectures, including taking lecture notes; what sort of books to use and how to learn from them, through effective note taking, reviewing your learning and testing yourself, how to sift out the rubbish from the Internet and search effectively using IT, making the most of the library and how to find appropriate review articles from journals that give the most up to date view.

In the chapters on *Learning Clinical Skills* and *Clinical Communication Skills*, we offer guidance on how to be self-directed in learning these skills, how to make the most out of simulation and how to capitalise on the richness that learning with patients offers. We specifically cover the clinical learning environment, as many students find the clinical setting (hospital wards, general practice) a very different and unstructured environment to learn in, we discuss how to get the most from your clinical tutors and where some of the hidden learning opportunities are. The ward round as a learning opportunity gets a special mention. With respect to clinical communication skills, we present an evidence-based approach and advice on learning both in simulation and in the clinical environment: learning both by doing and also by watching others. New in the second edition, we highlight the role of empathy and the ways in which diversity affects our practice and include a new section on how to give information effectively. We discuss the essential nature of feedback, both how to give effective feedback and also how to receive it, and how to act on it. Finally, we cover the patient presentation, a common cause of anxiety among both medical students and their supervisors. Throughout both chapters, we make no apologies for repeatedly stressing the primacy of patient care.

Much of the learning in medical schools in the United Kingdom is through *Working in a Group*. Working and learning in a group is inescapable in medicine and this section starts with a discussion on the pros and cons of group work and how to get the best from it. It specifically discusses Problem-Based Learning (PBL) and its variants, informal learning groups and how to make interprofessional learning work.

Students at medical school often struggle with developing an *Academic Writing* style, referencing appropriately and concepts of plagiarism. We give an introduction to these areas in a dedicated chapter, which we hope will start you off with safe foundations.

Portfolios and Reflection are inescapable in undergraduate and postgraduate medical education, and the chapter on the subject provides a pragmatic overview on what portfolios are, how to make them work for you and demystifies some of the concepts of reflection.

For the rest of your life, there will be too much to do at work and too much to do at home. Balancing social and professional lives forms a recurring theme in research about stress in doctors. The chapter on *Life – Work Balance* provides some guidance into how to manage both a healthy social life and a healthy study life and, most importantly, will help you get into good habits right at the start of your professional career. Both time management and stress management are covered here.

The chapter on *Revision* builds on and summarises the principles from the previous ones, discussing how to manage the learning environment, prioritising, planning and timetabling and managing stress. This chapter, above all others, offers wholesome, sensible advice on how to manage the limited time running up to exams.

The chapters on *Exam Technique* cover generic advice about how to approach exams, lists the different kinds of assessments that you might face at medical school and then offers specific advice on how to make the most from each of these. It includes how to do your best in multiple-choice, extended matching question exams, data interpretation questions and how to survive the OSCE or clinical skills exam. We discuss coping mechanisms that do not work, alongside those that do and advice on how to manage exam stress. New in this edition is specific advice on the latest trend in assessment – the dreaded 'Situational Judgement Test' (SJT) – which should help you prepare effectively and recognise what the questions are actually looking for.

Increasingly, medical students are involved in formal and informal teaching of others. The new chapter on *Teaching, Mentoring and Coaching* helps guide you through this, linking clearly from the chapters on how students learn, in order to explain how you can help others learn.

In this second edition, we provide a new chapter on *Professionalism*. Professionalism is the very foundation of medical practice and this is mirrored throughout this book. Professionalism is not separate, but integrated within each chapter. Whether it be learning effectively, encouraging life-long learning, concepts of referencing and plagiarism or a strong emphasis on learning in order to provide excellent care for patients, rather than to pass exams, you will find little in this book that will not count towards your developing professionalism. What this chapter specifically covers is how to learn professionalism, how it is assessed and some of the dilemmas around professionalism, particularly the quagmire that is digital professionalism. We hope that this chapter will help you to review and actively manage your 'digital footprint'. In addition, it may stimulate you to become involved with this emerging, rapidly changing field.

Finally, the chapter on *Thinking Ahead: Selected Study Components, Careers and Electives* offers some thoughts about longer term planning of learning – including which optional components of your course to choose, which electives to go on and some discussion on how to check out which career in medicine might be right for you.

How to use this book

This book has been written to provide a whole view, but each chapter has been designed to stand alone, with considerable cross referencing. Whether you prefer to start at the beginning and read start to finish or dip in and out, both approaches will work. We highly recommend that you read with some rough paper handy and *actively engage* with the few exercises that you will find in most chapters – it will be easy to skip them, but your understanding and learning will not be as deep if you do. Teaching on learning styles (what kind of learner are you) and on life – work balance is often unappealing. We have worked hard to make these chapters relevant, interesting and practical; they are fundamental and we would strongly encourage you to give them a go.

Summary

This book will not teach you what you need to know to be a doctor. However, by using this book actively you *will* learn how to study more effectively and efficiently at medical school, how to balance studying with an enjoyable social life and how to show your best abilities in the exams. In other words, this book will show you not only how to survive but also how to *thrive* at medical school and how to enjoy learning for the rest of your life.

Chapter 1 **What kind of learner are you?**

OVERVIEW

This chapter forms a foundation for the rest of this book. It will help you become aware of your learning preferences and the factors that tend to affect your learning. This awareness itself will be useful to you, both with respect to planning your learning and with respect to highlighting which chapters of the book you are likely to find particularly important. We have tried to give a brief overview of the most important factors and have tried to encourage you to make some judgements. You might want to revisit this chapter when you have finished the book to see if your impressions have changed.

Introduction

This chapter might be quite tough to work through. It asks you to take time away from reading to think about the things that affect your learning. The temptation will be just to read on; however, you will benefit considerably from having a few sheets of paper handy and trying to answer each question. Concentrate on each brief exercise and answer it as best you can, it will make the information sink in much better. At the end of the chapter, we have put a summary diagram, which we hope will highlight where you have assessed your strengths and weaknesses.

We will cover the following aspects of learning:

- cognitive aspects (how **deep** is your learning?)
- motivation (what **drives** you to learn?)
- self-regulation of study skills (are you **aware** of how you learn?)

How to Succeed at Medical School: An Essential Guide to Learning, Second Edition. Dason Evans and Jo Brown.
© 2015 John Wiley & Sons, Ltd. Published 2015 by John Wiley & Sons, Ltd.

- how do you know when you know enough?
- conception of learning (what you think learning is for?)
- learning in groups (love it or hate it)
- mood and learning (a help or a hindrance)
- VARK (your preferences in using your senses in learning).

You may want to have a brief break after each section, as there is quite a bit to think about.

Aspects of learning

You may have already completed learning style inventories or psychometric tests to try and define what sort of learner you are. There are all sorts of different learning styles and each tends to look at slightly different aspects of learning. The authors of the learning styles inventories claim that greatness can be reached by understanding how you think and learn, using their learning style inventory of course. Our aim is more modest – we hope that by thinking about how you learn, you will become aware of what aspects of learning you will find easier and where the challenges might lie ahead for you.

Filling in a learning style questionnaire was fantastic, it helped me realise the kind of learner I am and build on my natural style.

Jo, first-year graduate entry student.

Cognitive aspects

This refers to the way that you go about building new information into memories – how much do you skim over the surface or how much do you struggle to really understand? How well can you remember something that you have learned? For how long?

EXERCISE

Think about a topic that you learnt really well. How 'deep' was your learning? How much did you think about how your new learning linked in to what you knew already? Did you learn to understand or did you learn to memorise? Which do you find easier?

Make a judgement call, on the line below. Where would you put yourself?

I tend to try and memorise facts, and try not to expend too much information on thinking about the application or understanding of what I'm learning.

I prefer to learn to understand, I link new knowledge to old knowledge, I think I'm a deep learner.

If you have a preference for memorisation (the left-hand end of the line), then you will do very well with some things – drug names, anatomy, tests that ask you to regurgitate facts – but you are likely to struggle more on those tasks that require a deep understanding or application of the facts; unfortunately, a good amount of research indicates that students scoring towards the right tend to do better at medical school. You might think about some strategies to encourage you to shift more to the right, and in Chapter 2 (*Learning Knowledge*), we will go through some of these. If you tend to memorise as many facts as possible shortly before exams, forgetting them shortly after and have an easy time the rest of the year, then you will run into trouble with the volume of work in medicine and will need to start working regularly; this might be a challenge for you.

We give more tips on encouraging deep learning in Chapter 2, and advice on timetabling and regular study in Chapter 8.

Motivation

What makes you learn? Do you learn for interest, or perhaps to pass exam or even to please others? Some medical students learn best because they are fascinated by the science of medicine, others learn best when they can see the practical application of their learning and a few learn best when someone is standing over them pressurising them.

EXERCISE

Spend a minute thinking about what motivates your learning. You might want to spend some time talking with your friends about this, be honest with yourself. As you come to a decision, think about how you might make use of this insight.

I am most motivated to learn by:

- If you find the **science fascinating**, spend a couple of hours each week in the library looking at the journals – *Nature*, The *Lancet*. When learning about diabetes, you will want to read about insulin receptors, about the pathology, about the underlying mechanisms by which diabetes causes increased cardiovascular risk, in addition to the core areas that you *need* to learn. The commonest pitfall if you are this kind of learner is that you might have some trouble with knowing when to stop reading and when enough is enough – you cannot have a PhD level of knowledge on everything in medicine; we discuss tactics to manage this in Chapter 2.
- If it is patients and the **practical application of knowledge** that does it for you, you might find some of the bookwork in medicine rather dull and difficult to digest. Spend time thinking about practical applications. If you are learning about dry biochemical pathways, read also about clinical presentations of patients with problems in those pathways. You can look for case studies or even patient videos online that are relevant to your learning. You will want to buy some clinical textbooks early, so that you can read around clinical features of diseases. When learning about the pathology of the cervix, have a read about cervical smears, about the diagnosis and treatment of cervical cancer, think about how what you are learning will affect the care you give to patients. You might ask a friendly gynaecologist if you can sit in on their colposcopy clinic. See as many patients as possible and read about the conditions that you have seen – you will remember information much more clearly if you can link it in your memory to a patient you have seen.
- Many students are most highly **motivated by exams**. If this is you, then look up the exam structure early in the year – look at the objectives, plan how you will cover them. Use past questions to structure your learning and to test yourself, write your own, learn in a group and write tests for each other. The revision section of this book will appeal to you (Chapter 9) and also some of the study strategies in Chapter 2.

- Does **'knowing that you've done a good job'** motivate you to learn more? For many of us, praise and reward are important. If it is a major driver for you, you might want to be pragmatic in some of your learning. If you are sitting in an asthma clinic next Thursday, then learn about the management of asthma before then. You will feel like you understand what is going on, you will ask sensible questions and the clinician in clinic is likely to be impressed – this will motivate you to study more. This simple technique works exceptionally well!
- There are a few students who thrive on **external pressure**. They love teachers who intimidate students, whereas most of their peers tend to hide in threatening environments, they thrive in them. If this is you, then you might want to try and create situations that will drive you to learn. Agree deadlines with tutors or your peers, agree to teach students in your year or the year below; encourage them to try and catch you out, so that you know that you will have to learn your topic well.

Of course, you will not fit singly into any one of these five vignettes, but you will know which ones apply most to you. You are also likely to find that different topics might have different motivations for you. Clearly, there will not be a single strategy that applies to you. You cannot only read about the conditions that you have seen patients with or you will never learn about the rare ones. Similarly, if you are 100% examination focused, you might miss out on the things that are important but not examined. However, knowing and manipulating what motivates you in order to maximise your study is a key skill. It might even be worth pinning a note up on the wall above your desk, reminding you of what motivates you.

Self-regulation of study skills

Students who are aware of how they are learning (this is called metacognition) tend to perform much better than those who do not. This book is largely about helping you develop effective study skills and an awareness of when and how to use which ones. How aware of your learning are you? How consciously do you make choices in how you learn? Did you use different methods to learn different topics at school? If not, why not? The more you can learn to think about *how* you are learning, the more you will develop as an effective learner.

EXERCISE

Think about the following tasks. Spend 2 minutes on each task thinking about how you would go about it. Time yourself; it will be time well spent.

- You have a list of complications of diabetes to learn.
- You have to memorise a list of drug names for treating high blood pressure; the names all sound rather foreign to you.
- You have to learn the surface markings of the various lobes of the lungs so that you know which one is where when you are examining a patient.
- You have to learn how to take blood.

How easy was it to plan how you would go about each task? Was your plan for each task different or the same? Did you have several options for each task or just one? The more options and the more active your decisions, the easier you will find learning. If you tended to think of just one method of learning ('I would just keep repeating it until I remembered' or 'I would just learn it'), then you are likely to benefit from spending extra time on Chapter 2 and it might be worthwhile finding out if there are some study skills workshops run by your university. Improving in your study skills is an investment that will really pay off.

> *Learning how to learn was the most important thing I got from medical school, unfortunately I didn't realise this until the second year!*
>
> Rebecca, finalist.

How do you know that you know enough?
The A-level syllabus that you studied was well defined, in terms of both breadth of topics and depth that you need to go to in each topic. This is not so true at medical school and, as we have already mentioned, knowing when to stop can be a challenge. Some students are excellent at monitoring their progress and use the sort of tricks that we discuss in the chapter on learning knowledge (Chapter 2), but others either tend to learn far too much (and run out of time) or learn far too little.

EXERCISE

Think for a minute how you know when you have learnt enough on a topic. What evidence do you use that you know something?

This evidence that you rely on to know that you know enough on a topic may be objective, subjective or 'non-evidence'. **Objective measures** might include testing yourself from a book of past questions, or writing questions before you start learning from the course objectives and seeing if you can answer them when you think that you have finished learning; perhaps you try and explain it to someone else and see if you can answer all their questions. More **subjective evidence** will include others telling you that you are knowledgeable or perhaps you make a judgement that you can now understand something that previously you found rather complex, perhaps you look at the learning objectives and make a judgement on whether you have covered them. **Non-evidence** tends to be pretty useless, it includes judgements such as judging the number of hours that you have looked at a page, or how many books you have on the subject or how tidy your notes look as some 'guesstimate' of how much you have learnt.

You are likely to use a blend of these three approaches, and students who tend to cross-reference objective and subjective measures are likely to have a far more accurate idea of where they are up to in their learning. Students who use non-evidence tend to be rather surprised when they fail exams – 'but I spent hours looking at the books' or 'but my notes are always so perfect'.

Conception of learning

What is learning for? What is learning about? Do you see learning as a passive increase in knowledge or perhaps as memorisation of facts; perhaps you see learning as a way of gaining information that you can apply in practice or perhaps you learn in order to try and make sense of the world around you. Students who tend to try and make personal meaning out of what they learn seem to be more motivated and achieve deeper learning.

You might have left secondary school thinking that learning was about getting facts into your head. If so, you should be aware of the transition in higher education, where you will be expected to question, debate and weigh up different, conflicting evidence in order to try and make some sort of sense of the information in front of you and how it relates to the world around you. You can speed that transition by questioning yourself: asking 'What if … ?' or 'Why … ?' and 'What use is this information?'.

As an example, when you are learning about diabetes, you might ask yourself 'what if diabetes was not a disease that either you had or you did not have, but a continuum between normal blood sugar and damagingly high blood sugar?' Perhaps you will ask 'why is the threshold for diagnosing diabetes a fasting sugar of 7.0 mmol/L and not 7.4 mmol/L?' If you have a very concrete idea of facts, valid questions like these might be uncomfortable. It is better to have this discomfort and learn to manage it early on, rather than later in your career. You might have to trust us on this one!

Learning in groups

Collaborative learning has its pros and cons. Some students feel that they can only really learn through discussion and debate with others and they tend to struggle to find people with whom you can discuss everything that you have learnt. If this is you, you will benefit from reading the chapters on study skills (Chapter 2) and revision (Chapter 9). In contrast, some students find that they hate to study with others. These students tend to struggle to know whether they are learning to the right depth and they really struggle with clinical and communication skills learning, as feedback from peers and peer practice is crucial. If you fit into this group, the chapters on clinical and communication skills learning (Chapters 3 and 4) and working in a group (Chapter 5) will be particularly relevant to you.

Mood

Mood affects learning. Have you ever been so angry or frustrated that you were unable to study? Or so passionate about a subject that everything you read seemed to make sense? 'Feeling' can be intimately involved with 'thinking'?

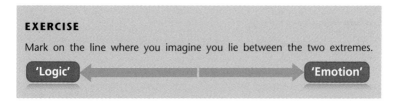

EXERCISE

Mark on the line where you imagine you lie between the two extremes.

'Logic' ⟵――――――⟶ 'Emotion'

Are there things that particularly swing you one way or another along this line? Some people find certain triggers throw them into emotional responses; guilt, for example, drives some to study but handicaps others. How about anxiety? Do you spend too much time worrying about the things you have not done rather than getting on and doing them?

What if you are on the other end of the scale, emotion never affects your thinking and learning, would you be missing out on the passion, the buzz of knowing that you are 'on a roll'? How will you develop empathy if you cannot see how emotion affects people's decisions (logically, surely everyone should agree to take part in medical research)? What about teamwork skills – how will you relate to others if you cannot see the emotional contexts in which they exist?

Think about where you are on the line and consider at what point on that line you might be more productive. Spend some time considering how you can actively manage the triggers and swings to be a little more productive a little more of the time. We have worked with many students and the simplest strategies are usually the best – a young woman whose studying used to be distracted by regular family crises moved out of home. When phone calls replaced knocks on her bedroom door, she discovered that she could switch off her phone while she was studying and she could study with a clear head.

Sometimes emotion clouds *all* your thoughts, and that is a time to get help. Indeed, everyone will struggle with the way that they are feeling and the way that affects their work at one time or another in their careers. In Chapter 8, we talk about avenues to ensure that you gain support when you need it.

VARK: using your senses

Think about incense. What comes immediately to mind? For some people they will see something relating to incense – perhaps the smoke curling up from a burning pot. Others will hear something – perhaps the ringing noise that an incense burner in church makes when it is swung or the word incense being said. Others might see the word as it is written, perhaps think about the different meanings of the word: 'pieces of fragrant substance' or 'to infuriate'. Finally, you might think about the movements that you would make to light or to swing the incense around.

It seems that some people have a visual preference, others an auditory or aural preference. Some prefer to read or write things to learn them and others have a strong kinaesthetic preference – that is physically to do things. The VARK learning style has come up for criticism, but it has some uses. Look at the following descriptions and think of how much they each apply to you.

Visual people will like to use colour and shapes, and they draw flow charts and like to have everything in sight in front of them. They like books that are visually appealing, with small blocks of text, plenty of tables and diagrams. They might find learning visual topics like anatomy much easier than memorising lists of words.

Aural people like to listen, they think that lectures are better than books and like it when someone explains things to them in words or they explain to others. They remember the anecdotes from the lecture, or what that patient said and sometimes they forget to write things down as they are too busy listening. They are not fond of books and tend to read books by forming the words in their heads. Sometimes their lips move when they are reading.

Those with a **read/write preference** tend to like books and texts and lists. They might copy out chunks of text from the book to form their notes, which are often quite lengthy and quite dry. They are good at spelling and can remember lists of words. They might look at a foreign word and work out what it means from similar words that they know.

Kinaesthetic learners like to learn by doing. They like practical applications – 'this goes there'. Real-life examples are great and learning by trial and error really consolidates their learning. Abstract things are more difficult for them and they strive to think of applications for what they are learning.

EXERCISE

For each of these preferences, rate whether you think that you are strong (you often think and learn in this way), average (you sometimes think and learn in this way) or weak (you rarely think or learn in this way)

	Weak	Average	Strong
Visual learning			
Aural/auditory learning			
Read/write learning			
Kinaesthetic learning			

Most people have a preference: some have strong preferences, others have a more even spread.

Think about your preferences, your strengths. This will give some indication of the sorts of tasks and subjects that you will find easiest. Think about how you can capitalise on your strengths:

- If you are a visual person, are you making best use of colour and pictures? Would you be better making your notes on a pad of A3 rather than A4 so that you can see more in one glance? Do you take one of those 4- or 10-colour pens into lectures with you? If not, why not? Do you try and convert difficult concepts into flow charts or cartoons? You will like the section on concept mapping in Chapter 2.
- If you are an auditory person, then do you make the best use of lectures, sitting near the front, away from distractions? Have you tried using tapes or reading your notes out loud? Do you ever put difficult facts to music to help you remember? You will find teaching and explaining to others really useful. How about starting a study group or a debating society?

- If you like the written word, you can write brief descriptions of diagrams or flow charts. You can change the words that your notes are written in, choosing your own words, so that you are sure that you are processing the information. You can write down patient stories, make lists and write essays. You might well like studying in libraries. Perhaps you could start an online group with others from your medical school or other medical schools where you explain things to each other on a message board or wiki.
- If you have a kinaesthetic approach, you will want to find practical applications for what you are learning. Get out there and do things – if you have seen a patient with a diabetic foot ulcer you will find it much easier to read about it. Apply what you have learned whenever you can, search for relevance. Use your imagination and imagine things happening when you read about them.

Think also about your weaknesses and how you can address them. There are two main approaches here. First you can try and redesign the task to play to your preferences. If you have to memorise a list of drug names and you are terrible at 'read/write' but strong on auditory memory, make up a song or a poem and sing it out loud. If you have a preference for visual things, turn the words into pictures: the drug zopiclone might become a number of identical (clones) Z-shaped floppy aliens (zoppy), all sleepy in bed (zopiclone is a sleeping pill).

The second way that you might address your weaknesses is to train yourself to be stronger in these areas. Timetable extra time for the tasks that you might find challenging, and ask your peers what tricks they use. You can find others with similar preferences to you (the incense exercise is a good one, although lots of people say 'the smell', which does not fit well into VARK, but is discussed more in Chapter 9) and find out how they learn. If, as a group, you all hate learning vocabulary then at least you can empathise when you are testing each other on drug names – you will most likely learn at a similar rate.

You can find out more about VARK at www.vark-learn.com or by typing VARK into your favourite Internet search engine. There is not a huge amount of evidence for VARK over any of the other dimensions of learning listed above but, like the others, it is useful to help you think about where your strengths and weaknesses lie, how you can capitalise on your strengths and actively manage your weaknesses.

Learning styles

As we mentioned at the start of this chapter, different learning style inventories tend to measure different combinations of the aspects of learning

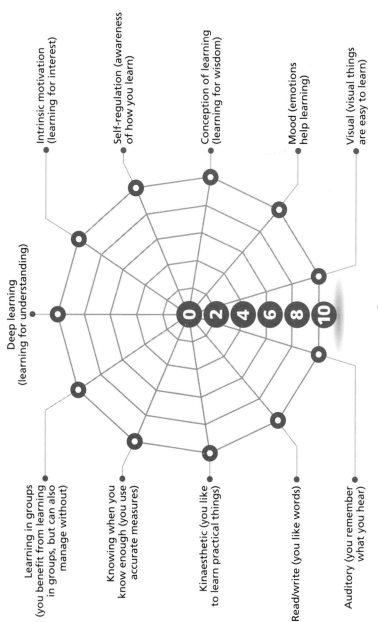

Figure 1.1 Summary.

that we have listed. If your medical school has a progressive curriculum, you might well fill out a questionnaire on your learning style and even get some numbers or a graph that will summarise your preferences. We would recommend that you look through this chapter a couple of times and actually do the exercises and answer the questions. Write some notes on where you identify your strengths and weaknesses, triggers that upset your learning and tips that maximise your learning.

Summary

This chapter has asked you to make multiple judgements about factors that affect your learning, which is not something you might have done before. Your judgements might not have been terribly accurate and we would recommend that you revisit this chapter again when you have read the remainder of the book and had a chance to think in more depth about what factors affect your learning.

The multiple aspects within this chapter have made it rather complex. You might find Figure 1.1 useful in summarising the chapter – you can mark on each axis where you think your strengths are (perhaps you decide 10 relates to "strength" or "no problem").

References and further reading

Coffield, F. (2004a). *Learning Styles and Pedagogy in Post-16 Learning: A Systematic and Critical Review*. London, Learning and Skills Research Centre.
Coffield, F. (2004b). *Should We be Using Learning Styles?: What Research has to Say to Practice*. London, Learning and Skills Research Centre.

Questions and answers

Q: I have done an online test for VARK and my kinaesthetic score is low – will I have trouble learning clinical skills?

A: The predictive validity of these different tests is not great. Some studies have suggested that students with either deep (learn to remember and understand) or pragmatic (learn to pass exams effectively) learning styles do better in medical school exams than those with superficial styles (cram facts for the exams, skim over the top), but this really is not rocket science to understand. The usefulness in these inventories is that they encourage you to think about your preferences and the way that you tend to learn – do you think that this judgement is true for you? If you tend to avoid practising when learning a skill, how are you going to make sure that you practise your clinical skills a great deal when you are learning them? See Chapter 3 for an in-depth description of effective clinical skills learning.

Q: My medical school not only makes me do learning style inventories, but also inventories on how I work in a team – it drives me mad!

A: There are inventories for almost everything you can imagine, as a significant proportion of the world is made up of people who like to measure things, everything; in fact they even make up new things in order to measure them. As you might guess from this chapter, our emphasis is less on formal, accurate, statistically significant measurement, but much more on using these tools pragmatically in order to develop your self-awareness. We know that students who develop self-awareness with respect to learning outperform their peers, so see what you can take out from the exercises. Perhaps you want to find Professor Coffield's papers (Which critiques, and criticises, learning styles inventories in depth) and engage in a discussion with your course convenor.

Chapter 2 **Learning knowledge**

OVERVIEW

This chapter introduces some of the key issues and strategies for learning knowledge. We discuss the different types of knowledge and tips for improving your learning based on what we know about how memory works. Finally, we discuss different learning environments and how to make best use of them.

Introduction

There is one thing that we can be pretty sure about – that you are intelligent. You did well at school (you might even have been near the top of the class) and some of you will have relied on a good memory, but not a great deal of study, to pass your exams. Unfortunately, medical school is not like secondary school, college or sixth form. The curriculum is not as clearly set as for A-levels, and it has a tendency to change a little while you are still trying to follow it. The volume of work is huge, too big for even the best minds to hold without effort and too much information to cram into your head the week before the exam. The source of knowledge might be different too: you might have been told what to learn at school – learn the classes and do the set homework and you will do well at most secondary schools. In medicine, you will not get taught everything that you need to know, and yet you will still be expected to learn it – to work out what you need to learn, to work out ways of learning it, to work out ways of knowing when you have learnt it and to get on and learn it.

This drastic change of emphasis comes as a culture shock to many. This chapter highlights some of the issues with learning in medical school and looks to established theories from educational psychology and established

How to Succeed at Medical School: An Essential Guide to Learning, Second Edition.
Dason Evans and Jo Brown.
© 2015 John Wiley & Sons, Ltd. Published 2015 by John Wiley & Sons, Ltd.

study skills techniques to make your learning as efficient and effective as possible.

There are some key messages running through this chapter, which might be worth highlighting here.

- The purpose of learning is to be able to recall and apply information; therefore, it makes sense to learn it in a way that will make recall and application easier.
- Learning is an active process – if you are not engaged with the material that you are learning, then you will not be learning.
- Learning to learn effectively and efficiently, like any other skill, requires deliberate and reflective effort over time. If you want to learn a new way of learning, it will take 3 months, or so, of practice before you become fluent. If you invest time and effort now, these skills will stay with you and help you for the rest of your life.
- There is no end to what you *could* learn in medicine, so you will need to learn what is important and when you can tell that you know enough about a subject.
- The only way to survive the load of learning at medical school is through regular, active, self-directed learning. It is probably possible to pass the exams in the first 2 years of most curricula by cramming if you have a good memory, but it will not be possible after this, and your knowledge will be seriously deficient. Start studying for being a doctor from week 1 of your course.
- Spend time not only thinking about *what* you are learning but also *how* you are learning – what works for you? What works for this task? How could you improve your learning?
- Learning in medicine is a lifelong process, medical school is just the start, and you might as well try and get the foundations right.

How do I know what to learn?

Medical education is unlike other types of higher education. Medicine has no start and no end, and it is close to impossible to define exactly the knowledge, skills and attitudes that are required to be a doctor. Medicine is rapidly changing, so by the time you get to the end of a 4-, 5- or 6-year curriculum, exactly what you need to be able to know and to be able to do will have changed. Understandably, students struggle and stress trying to find out what they are expected to know, and this section aims to give some pointers on how to find out. The bad news is that there is not one published list of what is needed to make a good doctor, but the good news is that there are plenty of pointers out there. You will need to make some judgements about what you want and need to learn. For the rest of your professional life you will need to make those same judgements, so it is not a bad habit to get into.

Your medical school is likely to publish a curriculum listing core required knowledge in one form or another (perhaps as a list of core conditions), and this should provide you with some guidance. It might change, and more importantly it might not reflect what you need to know to be a safe and effective doctor, so you will need to spend some time considering what else you should know, and to what depth. Textbooks are handy, looking through the table of contents of a medium-sized core text will give you a good idea, as will looking through the index of some thin undergraduate books. You might want to look at both clinical books and basic science books (anatomy, pathology, physiology etc.), as you will be expected to learn hard science and its clinical application.

Self-directed versus teacher-directed learning

In some secondary schools, the teaching is excellent. You were taught what you needed to know to do well in your exams. Learn your lessons, do your set-work well and you did well in your GCSEs and in your A-levels. Medicine (and indeed most higher education) is different. You will need to learn to take control of your own learning; after all, this is how you will be learning for the rest of your professional life as a doctor. Keep a notebook or a section of your diary where you can jot down things you want to look up and set aside regular time to do so. These might be things that you think are important for exams or for your practice as a doctor or they might be things that you find interesting and might make you a more rounded doctor.

Just learning the taught components of your course and doing the set assignments will not be enough to become a good doctor.

> I prefer to be taught things and have always gone to teachers to find things out. It was a real culture shock at my medical school when they just replied 'how are you going to look that up?' Sometimes I wish they would just teach me.
>
> Catriona, first-year medical student.

Binge learning versus regular learning

There is no way of escaping it, and you will need to develop a habit of regular self-directed learning. Our Chapter 8 on *Life–Work Balance* covers this in more depth. You might in the past have crammed for exams, and your memory might be such that you can memorise a whole lot of facts and hold them in your memory for a week or two. There are three problems with doing this in medicine. First, the volume of facts will become too great to hold; at some point, you will not be able to manage, and at that point, you will realise that you are actually years behind in your knowledge. Second, you will not be asked to just regurgitate facts, instead you will be asked to apply knowledge: you need a deep level of understanding to be able to do this, and cramming does not give you that kind of level.

Finally, and most importantly, you are not studying to pass exams; you are studying to be a doctor. Cramming information in your head just before an exam and forgetting it shortly after will not help you care for patients, regardless of whether you passed.

You will need a diary and a timetable, and you will need to plan regular self-directed learning, some of which will involve looking up new topics and some of which will involve reviewing your previous learning to consolidate it into long-term memory (more on this later in the chapter). If you get into good habits early in the course, they will pay major dividends during the course and long after.

Lifelong learning and continuing professional development

The phrase, lifelong learning, is a bit of a mantra in higher education and gets brought out at every opportunity. Skipping all the rhetoric, as a doctor you need to continue learning, all the time, day in day out for the rest of your professional life. For the vast majority of the time, no-one will tell you what you need to learn. You will need to know what you do know (relatively easy), know what you do not know (which is harder), prioritise what you need to know, or what you might need to know (difficult if you have a tendency to be indecisive), work out a way of learning it (bad news, plenty of studies show that exotic conferences are a terrible way of learning) and work out a way of knowing when you know enough on that topic and can move on (Figure 2.1). Appraisals, some curricula, your mentors and drug representatives touting their wares might all help you, but the emphasis will always come down to you.

One of your aims at medical school has to be to learn how to learn, and learn how to continue to learn, to keep up to date. It is daunting, but actually it is fun too.

Depth versus breadth

Here is a key issue that students struggle with. One student we worked with had a tendency to always study to far too great a depth. She was working with a group of others close to finals and they agreed to go away and study liver

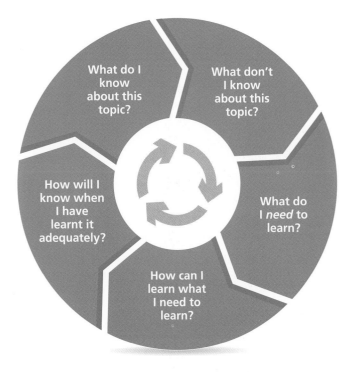

Figure 2.1   Planning self-directed learning.

disease over the next 2 days and then come back and test each other. This student became lost in the molecular pathology of primary biliary cirrhosis, finding deeper and deeper books to go into and never got to read about gallstones. It would be possible to study for a PhD on the molecular pathology of this rare condition and still not understand it completely. As a doctor, it is not a condition that you are likely to see often (if at all), let alone need to know the molecular pathology of it. On the flip side of the coin, we have also seen plenty of students who do the opposite: they buy the thinnest books possible and can write two lines on any condition in medicine – only two lines though! (Figure 2.2).

Working out to what depth you need to learn is a difficult balancing act. You cannot and will not ever know everything and yet you probably want to know more than the minimum. Throughout the rest of this chapter, we try and give tips on different ways you might check that you are working to an appropriate depth.

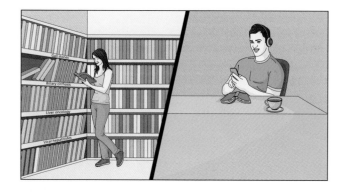

Figure 2.2   Finding the right depth to study can be difficult.

I really like to understand things fully. Sometimes I spend hours and hours on one small thing, looking in the library and on the net to try and understand it completely. I ran out of time in my revision and did badly in my first year exams – I think I've learnt my lesson.

Dimitris, second-year medical student.

One answer: Bloom's taxonomy

Benjamin Bloom made a name for himself leading a group of educational psychologists in an attempt to define different levels of knowledge, in order to guide students and their examiners. He defined seven levels of knowledge, which are often used religiously by educationalists (Table 2.1). As with any model, it is not perfect, but it is particularly useful to help you think about the purpose and the depth of knowledge that you are learning.

At medical school, you will be expected to learn knowledge at more than a basic level. You will be asked to apply your knowledge, use it to problem solve, use it to critique papers and use it to hypothesise and create new ideas – simply knowing and understanding will not be enough.

Imagine that you are seeing a person with diabetes who has quite poor blood glucose control. Being able to recite a memorised list of causes for poor diabetic control is not going to help you very much – you will need to be able to take that knowledge, apply it, investigate what is going on for the patient, hypothesise which causes are most likely, test those hypotheses one way or another and explain it all to the patient. Most of your exams will try and test these higher levels of knowledge, and when studying, you should use techniques to ensure that you are learning knowledge to this level, more of this comes later.

Table 2.1   Bloom's levels of knowledge

Knowledge (remember)	You know enough to be able to recite knowledge by rote (e.g. you can recite the 15 causes of clubbing)
Comprehension (understand)	You understand the knowledge, so can explain it to others (e.g. you can explain what clubbing is)
Application (apply)	You can use the knowledge you have to solve problems (you use your knowledge of clubbing to try and work out why the patient in front of you has clubbed fingers)
Analysis (analyse)	You can use the knowledge you have to compare and contrast with other knowledge and see how it fits in with other people's assumptions and/or hypotheses (e.g. compare and contrast type 1 and type 2 diabetes; compare and contrast the electron as a particle and the electron as an electromagnetic wave)
Synthesis (create)	You can use knowledge, integrated with other knowledge, to produce new hypotheses (e.g. you know glucose crosses the placenta and that insulin does not; you know that in diabetes glucose tends to run high, so you hypothesise that the baby of a woman with diabetes will produce high levels of insulin itself and so will be at risk of going 'hypo' after birth)
Evaluation (evaluate)	You use your knowledge to assess, critique or judge others

Adapted from Bruning, Schraw *et al.* (2004).

EXERCISE

Look at the following exam questions; to what level of Bloom's taxonomy do they assess knowledge?

Q1 The following are causes of clubbing (true or false).

Q2 A man presents with clubbing and jaundice, which of the following are likely diagnoses?

Q3 A man presents with clubbing and shortness of breath, which one of the following investigations would be most appropriate?

Q4 Critique the box (Figure 2.3) 'what is clubbing?' and use your knowledge to suggest improvements.

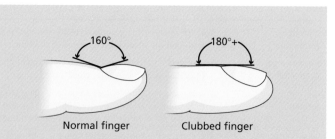

Figure 2.3 What is clubbing? Clubbing is a physical sign, a favourite of clinicians, where the bed of the nail is swollen, so that the finger nail or toe nail, rather than sliding downwards into the digit looks like it slopes in the opposite direction.

The mind, memory and learning

Without wishing to upset all those neurophysiologists and neuropsychologists, no one really seems to understand how memory works. There are a couple of theories though, borne out by experimental research, which do provide some pointers on how memory might work particularly on how to maximise learning.

Left brain, right brain

Positron emission tomography (PET) scans and functional magnetic resonance imaging (fMRI) scans as well as older electrophysiology work show that if you are right-handed, the left-hand side of your brain seems to relate to words, fact, logic, whereas the right-hand side deals much more with emotion, feelings and imagery. The theory goes that if you use both halves of your brain while learning, you are more likely to remember. This seems true: if you use as many senses and exaggeration and emotion when trying to learn something, you are more likely to remember it. One of the causes of clubbing is pus in the lungs (which occurs when there are lung abscesses, and conditions called empyema and bronchiectasis). If you visualise someone with hugely clubbed fingers, imagine pus dripping out from their lungs through their chest wall, dripping on the floor. It makes you feel sick, it is green and smelly, your imaginary person uses his or her clubbed *finger nails* to pick at the pus. Spend a moment imagining this (look up a picture of clubbing if needs be), run through all your senses and exaggerate them (what can you hear, smell, feel, taste and see?) and do the same with your emotions (perhaps you are afraid, or disgusted, you feel nauseous and so forth). If you hold this image in your head and revisit it once or twice, you will never forget pus in the lung as a cause of clubbing.

> *I really love using colour and pictures, I remember things so much better when I can see them.*
>
> Sian, third-year medical student

The vaccination model of memory

As a health-care professional, you will be vaccinated against hepatitis B. You will be given the first injection, and this will cause a minor immune reaction, your antibodies will rise and then fall. When given a second injection, your immune memory will be heightened and the same with the third. So with each injection, your immune response and immune memory is strengthened. Not only are several injections better than one injection for strength and longevity of immune memory, but the timing also seems important – one injection today and the second in 5 years' time, is likely to be pretty useless.

There are parallels with memory, of course. If you learn a list of causes of clubbing and do not look at it for a year, you will be lucky if you can remember it. If you learn it now, review it in 3 days', 3 weeks' and 3 months' time, you will probably remember it for life (the rule of threes). This is one of the reasons why most medical schools have exams frequently and each exam will often cover the content of the last exam, in addition to the learning you have done since then. This is to encourage you to revisit and review your learning on a regular basis.

This has some practical implications for studying. Use your diary or timetable (Chapter 8) to mark down review sessions – perhaps one evening a week. Use this time to review notes that you made this week, 3 weeks ago and 3 months ago. If you use active learning principles (see later), you will be able to review your notes quickly and efficiently and extend your memory of the topics far beyond your peers.

Semantic networks

One of the leading models of memory is that memories are encoded in networks. One item of knowledge is linked to other items of knowledge like some massive, messy spider's web, with knowledge sitting at intersections of the silk and the web representing the links. Clubbing links to what you know about the anatomy of the fingers and links to the possible diagnoses, each of which links to what you know about them. There is also probably now a link to a revolting image of pus.

Memory is, therefore, constructed by linking new learning with your prior knowledge (interestingly enough, even if your prior knowledge on the subject is rather poor) and the strength of a memory, or of learning, depends on the strength of those links. In turn, the strength of those links depends on how many times you use them.

As an example, another cause of clubbing is inflammatory bowel disease, particularly two conditions called Crohn's disease and ulcerative colitis. You could try and learn that as an isolated fact or you could link it in with what you know of bowel diseases. When you learn about causes of diarrhoea (such as Crohn's disease and ulcerative colitis), you think about the features you will look for on examination (such as clubbing), and when you read about the anatomy and histopathology of the bowel, you consider systemic manifestations of bowel disease (such as, you guessed it, clubbing), then that link between clubbing and inflammatory bowel diseases will be much stronger, and if you see a patient with clubbing, bowel disease will spring into your mind, similarly if you see a patient with Crohn's disease, you will know to look for clubbing.

The relevance for your learning is that when learning new things, always try and build links with what you know already, this will strengthen both the new learning and your prior knowledge.

Context is everything

In a rather elegant study in the 1970s, Godden and Baddeley investigated whether the physical context of learning affected the physical context of recall. They took scuba divers and taught them either on land or underwater and then tested them either on land or underwater. Participants who were tested in the same context as they learnt (land–land or underwater–underwater), did significantly better than participants who were tested in a different context than they learnt (land–underwater or underwater–land). The study was nicely controlled and is often quoted in educational literature. This sort of research lead to 'common sense' advice that you will find dotted through this book and particularly in the chapter on revision – practise for exams under exam conditions, consider using the same aromatherapy oils when studying as when being tested, learn with patients, from patients and for patients and learn for recall/for purpose. You might suggest that this sort of advice is rather a distant extrapolation from a study of scuba divers, but you would be wrong.

In 2010, educationalists (Finn *et al.*) at Durham Medical School published a similar piece of research, showing that medical students who learnt anatomy wearing scrubs performed better on a test when they wore scrubs rather than their usual clothes and students who learnt the same anatomy

Chapter 2

task in their usual clothes did better on a test when tested in these same clothes than in scrubs.

Thinking about the context of recall while you are learning is, therefore, important. It is one of the basic principles of active learning and modern approaches such as PBL (problem-based learning). When you learn anything, think about how, why and where you will be using that information.

For those of you who are fascinated by the effect of clothes on learning and behaviour, this in itself is a very new area of psychology and searching the Internet for 'enclothed cognition' will lead to some fascinating reading.

Active learning, passive learning

Have you ever seen someone asleep over (or under) a book? I have a fantastic picture of my brother asleep on the sofa with a copy of the *British National Formulary* (*BNF*) covering his eyes. We labelled it 'learning by osmosis'. Thinking about yourself, have you ever sat and stared at a page, read the same paragraph over and over before you realised that you had not taken in a word of it? We have seen plenty of students who sit and read books, look at the words, often spending many hours doing so, but then still do not seem to do well in the exams.

Effective learning is an active process requiring effort and energy. The volume of learning required in medicine is so much that even those with outstanding memories will not be able to just soak it all up and this will be a shock for many. Similarly, the fact that you will need to apply knowledge, will mean that those who try and just learn flat facts, to recall a paragraph or two of a core text, will have a lot of trouble taking that knowledge and using it in other contexts.

Tips for active learning

Before learning

- Ask questions – Why am I learning this? What will it tell me? How will I know when I have learnt it?
- Obtain an overview (look perhaps at the headings and subheadings in a text book).
- Write down what you know already on some rough paper, perhaps as a brainstorm or concept map (see later in the chapter).
- Write down some key questions that you should be able to answer at the end of your learning – perhaps use past exam questions.

During learning
- Do not write things down word for word, rather listen or read a section, and then write down what you think you need to know, in your own words.
- Write notes reliant on key words (see below).
- See where your learning links in with other things you know. Look at your brainstorm/concept map – is it right, what can you add to it?

After learning
- Tidy up your notes.
- Has your learning told you what you needed?
- Rewrite your network of key information.
- Can you put your notes away and answer those questions that you identified at the start?
- Can you explain what you learnt to someone else? Here is a great role play for a study group.

There are some tricks to make learning active; these principally revolve around the concept of **learning by doing**. For example, when making notes you can make them inn such a way that you have to engage with the material when you are making them, and also in such a way that will ensure that you engage with them when you review them rather than just read through them passively. We will discuss strategies for doing this in the next few sections. Whatever method you use, think about your learning and ensure that it is active learning.

Making notes

The key principle: keywords

Just about all effective note taking, whether from books or lectures, whether conventional or more modern approaches, depends on the concept of 'keywords'. A keyword is a word or short phrase that sums up a sentence or an idea. The keyword itself should remind you of the content of that sentence or idea and so keywords are personal – your keywords may not be the same as mine, depending on our different prior knowledge, although usually there is common ground. Keywords provide enough information to trigger recall. This paragraph can be summarised with the four keywords (OK, key phrases) represented in Figure 2.4.

If you look at these keywords after reading the previous paragraph, you should be able to recall what it was about. I have not included 'word or short

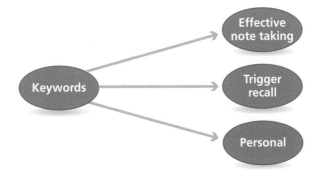

Figure 2.4 Key phrases.

phrase' as I know that about keywords already. Notice that if you had not read that paragraph, the keywords might not be that useful ('personal' could mean any number of things), so keywords aid recall of something that you have read or heard, but are not that useful as a starting point. Books of lists are popular with medical students, and these are basically someone else's lists of keywords. Trying to memorise these lists really does not help learning, despite whatever the introduction to the book says!

Where keywords come into their strength is when you have made them yourself. You can summarise and remind yourself of huge chunks of text books or lectures with one or two keywords and when revising and reviewing your notes these prompts should help you recall the main points. If they do not, you will need to glance at the book or lecture slides and you will very quickly say 'ah yes'.

If you are new to keywords, learning to make them can be quite difficult. You will need to practise and review how you are progressing on a regular basis. Start with texts and lectures that are not too heavy on facts and figures – clearly trying to make keywords from a book of lists would not be a good start. Try and summarise a chapter of this book with keywords, and then after a day, see if the keywords remind you enough of the content for you to explain it to someone else. Go back to the keywords that did not help and see if you need them or if you can rephrase them to work better for you. With a little practice, making keywords becomes second nature. For a book like this, a keyword or two for each paragraph is probably about right. This paragraph might be summarised by 'easy with deliberate practice', which reminds me not only that it is easy with practice, but also that practice is required and 'deliberate practice' to me means practice where I think about how I am learning while I practise.

SQ3R

The SQ3R is quite time-consuming if you do it properly and may be challenging if you have a high workload, but it does provide some good general principles for all note taking: – First **survey** the topic – have a look at reading lists, past exam papers, perhaps look at subheadings in a text book. Next **question** – why are you reading this? What do you want to get out of it? How will you know when you know enough? **Read** to understand, a paragraph at a time, without making notes. Next **re-read** to take notes and finally **review** whether the notes do the job.

This model encourages you to think actively about what you need to learn before you start making notes. It helps make your learning active, and provides you with structure in your learning. It should also help you to build new learning on top of your prior knowledge.

The Cornell method of taking notes

The Cornell method is a really simple modification of note taking, designed to make and subsequent reviewing of those notes into active learning. It was developed by Walter Pauk (from Cornell University, of course) in the 1950s, and it is now widely used internationally. The secret is in the preparation.

Before you start making notes, before the lecture or before you sit down with a book, take your blank paper and draw three lines. Draw a line across the top of the page so that you have dedicated space for a title (date, topic, other such information), draw a line across the page separating the bottom quarter – you will use this as a summary later – and finally draw a line down the left-hand side about 5 cm (2 inches) from the left. Write your notes in the main body of the page (the right-hand side).

After the lecture or when you close the book, look through your notes and tidy them up. Then on the left-hand column, write in the keywords or prompts or summary points that will help you recall the notes that you took. Finally, at the bottom of the page, write a one-sentence summary of what the page is all about.

This method is particularly useful in two respects. First it makes you review your notes and makes sure that you understand them. The reviewing, summarising and bringing out key concepts makes your learning active. The second thing it enables is easy, active revision. When revising just cover up the right-hand side of the notes with a piece of rough paper – look at each summary point on the left and write on the rough paper the details that link to that point. When you have done that for all the summary points, check your rough paper against the underlying notes, what is missing?

Of course, you can adapt the Cornell method to the task at hand and to your preferred learning. Perhaps you can use the summary space to write a handful of short answer questions, then when revising you can give them a go without looking at the notes and then look at the summary points in the cue column – do you want to add anything to your answers? Then look at the notes on the right – what did you leave out?

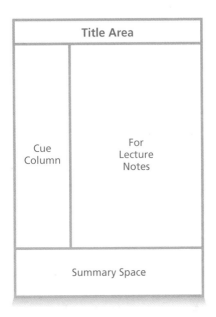

Concept mapping
The belief that knowledge is linked within memory makes the idea of concept maps rather appealing. Concept maps are diagrammatic representations of networks of related knowledge. Each node in a concept map is a keyword, and each linkage has a direction and an annotation that described the relationship between keywords. A concept map of this section so far might look something like Figure 2.5.

Concept maps are useful when there are complex interacting facts and to provide overviews of otherwise rather murky terrain. I know academics who keep all their references for academic papers in concept maps, so that they can see at a glance what papers to look for when researching a particular topic. You can draw concept maps by hand or use software for doing it. Generic software such as Microsoft PowerPoint and Word can build simple concept maps using the drawing and connector tools; there are also dedicated software

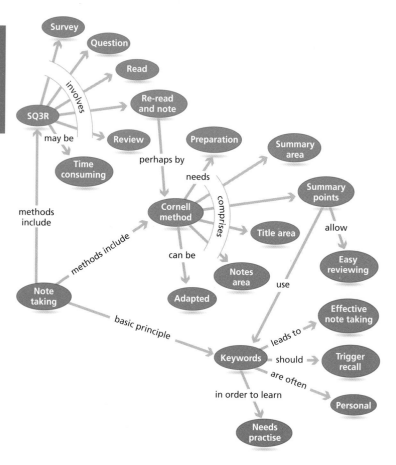

Figure 2.5 A concept map.

packages. Electronic concept maps are particularly useful for brainstorming as they allow you to rearrange concepts easily.

MindMaps

MindMaps, a term coined by Tony Buzan (1995), are a type of hier-archical concept map that makes use of colour and imagery (the right-brain–left-brain idea). They use keywords in a tree-like structure and encourage the writer to use as much of their imagery as possible. Figure 2.6 shows you one of two MindMaps I have written on note taking,

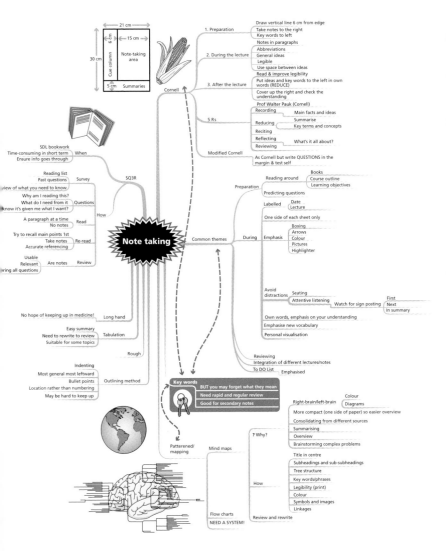

Figure 2.6 MindMaps.

the actual content is not important, but you can see the use of imagery (corn for Cornell, keys for keywords, etc.) that helps me remember the different areas and their content.

The main challenge in making MindMaps is that it is difficult to guess where to place the main stems – often you will find that you did not leave enough space for one or two of the sections. When making MindMaps from books, the general structure is reasonable to guess in advance from the subheadings and size of the various subsections. In lectures, this is trickier, although at the start of the presentation the lecturer might well give some structure ('Today I am going to cover three main aspects of diabetes'). Make your MindMap on A3 and do not get too stressed if you have to go onto another piece of paper. Spend 10 minutes at the end of the lecture or some other time that day in a spare moment to rewrite your MindMap as a best version – the rewriting will help it fit more logically to the page and will help you review what you learnt. You might decide that you do not need everything that you wrote down or that there is an area that looks a bit sparse and might need some additional bookwork to fill out.

MindMaps are personal things. They are best handwritten and annotated. Use colours and images that mean something to you. When revising, take a blank sheet of paper and see how much you can draw out again, then look at your original map and see what you missed. Use active techniques to revise; there is too much on a complex MindMap for you to learn just by looking at it. Similarly there are books of MindMaps for medicine that you can buy. These are usually little more than lists arranged in a tree structure. The key benefits of MindMaps for learning are first that you learn by creating them, by colouring them and by thinking what images might help you remember and second that they are personal to you.

Tony Buzan's book *Use Your Head* (1995) gives an excellent general guide to learning, and covers MindMaps in a lot more detail.

Cue cards

You can buy various size cue cards from most stationers. These are perfect if you tend to feel overloaded when revising. Make summary notes on to cue cards – one card one topic. Imagine a card on myocardial infarction: it could include key words summarising features on history, examination, special investigations, treatment, complications and pathology. You can carry it with you and try and remember what is on it in spare moments, and then check if you were right. You could do the same for many core conditions and either review them in turn or, when you are confident, choose one at random. Perhaps ask a friend to select a card at random and test you.

Tables

Constructing tables is a fantastic way of summarising data. Let's think about respiratory examination: there are 20 or so steps to the examination and 10 or so common clinical diagnoses, each with a different pattern of findings. Making a table with findings down one side and conditions across the top is great for highlighting the different findings between different conditions.

Making tables is very useful for summarising and understanding, but just looking at tables, perhaps in a book, is much less useful. Imagine the aforementioned example – it will have 200 bits of information in it – far too much to absorb by looking at it. If you want to revise a table, take a blank piece of paper and try and write it out again.

The right tools for the right job

You might be feeling frustration from this chapter – 'Hang on, which is the best way of making notes'? – the answer is very much 'It depends!' The best way depends on the task in hand (both the complexity and the environment) and your personal preference. For some tasks, Cornell will be the best option, and for others, a table might be best. If you are a visual person (see the section on learning styles, Chapter 1), then you might tend to have a preference for MindMaps, and if you are more of a words person, then you might lean more towards cue cards.

It is important to know that it takes up to 3 months to become slick at any new way of learning. If these aforementioned concepts are new to you, introduce them one at a time. Start with keywords and then when you are finding it easy to find the right keywords, perhaps try MindMaps or concept mapping for a couple of months. Keep a log of which methods seem to work for which tasks. Once you have mastered several methods, you will notice that you start using the most appropriate method automatically.

Learning environments

Learning from lectures

Some medical schools remain predominantly lecture based, whereas others use mostly small group work (Chapter 5). All schools will use lectures at one time or another and making the most out of them will help you a great deal.

Preparation is important, although many students find the organisation required challenging. Reading up on the topic before the lecture will help you understand the topic much more deeply. Imagine at the far extreme that you spent 20 minutes before the lecture making some notes on the topic of the lecture, using a leading text. You leave plenty of spaces in your notes and if there is anything that you do not understand after reading it twice, you just leave space. In the lecture, you sit back and listen, annotate your notes and fill in the gaps. You can work from your notes (as opposed to the lecturer's handouts, which are likely not to be in your style) and concentrate on understanding. You could prepare the night before or even get in a bit early and prepare over a coffee. Perhaps a more realistic alternative is that you spend 5 minutes the night before a lecture looking at the objectives of the lecture and then just scribbling down the main subheadings from the relevant section of a text book. That way you might well trigger some prior knowledge, and in the lecture, you will have a good idea of where the lecture is going.

> *I used to think that just 'being there' was enough, only when I talked to some friends after a lecture did I realise that I hadn't picked up as much as them.*

> Bruce, first-year medical student.

During the lecture make sure that all your papers are labelled clearly with the lecture and the date – you will thank yourself 6 months later when you drop your file and paper goes everywhere! Think about where you want to sit in the lecture theatre. Aim to sit somewhere where you will have to concentrate and where distractions will be at a minimum. If your friends tend to talk to you or distract you in other ways, save their company for the breaks and sit away from them in lectures. If they object, tell them that you must be stupid or something because you really need to concentrate hard to understand lectures. Buy them a coffee and they will forgive you!

Pay particular attention to the lecturer signposting important points or transitions between different parts of the lecture. Listen for 'importantly', 'don't forget', 'in summary', 'the (first, second, next etc.) key point that I want to make is ... ' and so on.

Write your notes in your own words and use keywords and bullet points as appropriate. Concentrate on writing down *your understanding* rather than the words on the slides. Use emphasis in your notes – boxes and arrows, pictures and colours. Highlight key points and ensure that the headings are clear. Box or circle any new words and their definitions.

After the lecture, tidy up your notes, think about how this lecture fits in with other learning that you have had. You might even combine several different lecture notes if there is substantial overlap – the importance is that you can understand and apply what you have learnt, not that you can regurgitate one particular lecturer's presentation.

Once in a while you will have a terrible lecture. It will be all over the place, hard to follow and it will come with a handout that has had all headings removed to save space. You will be tempted to spend hours trying to make sense of it all – do not bother. Look at the objectives for the lecture (the school will have published them somewhere) and just open an appropriate book. Imagine the clinical lecture on infertility was impossible to follow – just open a book on gynaecology for general practice and look at the infertility section, it will provide a good overview. When you understand the topic, if you really want to, then is the time to look back at the lecture. Hopefully, this would not happen often, but it is important to be aware that if you are finding a lecture impossible to follow, it might not be your fault and it might be a good indicator that you should use another source for your learning.

Learning from books

The same principles apply to learning from books as learning from lectures. Be attentive to your surroundings and possible distractions. If you are at home, turn the TV and radio off and put a do-not-disturb sign on the door. If you are working in the library, you might choose a seat that faces a wall to avoid watching the world go by.

It is probably best to make notes of one form or another, depending on the task in hand. Do not, whatever happens, just copy out chunks of text: unless you think about what you are reading, how will you learn it? Some people will just sit and read books, others annotate the pages (only if you own the book, please), but the trouble with that is that first the temptation is to think you are studying when you are, in fact, just looking at the page and, second, when you come to revise, you will have a whole mass of reading to do all over again. With deliberate, reflective practice, your notes should become a distillation of the key points, with an emphasis on the areas that you think are important and that you, personally, think that you might have difficulty remembering. In this way, your notes will be different from the books and will be different from another student's notes on the same subject.

As discussed previously, making notes is not good enough on its own, they need to be useful notes, you need to review them on a regular basis and when you review them you need to be learning actively (try to rewrite the key points, try to answer a couple of questions etc.).

Learning from the Internet

Here's an exercise: go to your favourite Internet search engine and type in 'Elvis is alive' or even 'Elvis is an alien' – if you use quotation marks it will only find that exact phrase. You will find plenty of evidence that it is true, Elvis *is* an alien (apologies to fans of the King). Similarly 'HIV is not sexually transmitted' and 'radiation is good for you'. The Internet is therefore full of misinformation, interspersed with some high-quality information. Working out which category the information you find fits into can be challenging.

Every medical student should receive training on finding reliable informa-tion on the Internet. If you have not, that is precisely the sort of request that will bring your medical librarian to tears of joy. There are some websites that give guidance on how to evaluate other websites for accuracy, one good one is QUICK: the 'quality information checklist' (which gives advice aimed at secondary schools, but is equally valid for the rest of us. Although the origi-nal website has ceased to exist, you can find the checklist mirrored on many other sites.) Another, www.discern.org.uk/, gives a questionnaire specifically aimed at evaluating health-related websites.

You will find some **portals**, websites that act as gateways to other high-quality sites: www.patient.co.uk, www.doctors.org, the student BMJ and BMA learning are just four of many examples. Websites that have a clearly described peer review process are likely to provide more reliable information than others.

Finding that review article

The web does, of course, provide a quick way of identifying high-quality arti-cles from peer-reviewed journals. Some of these articles may be of partic-ular use to you, and these will include educational articles and review arti-cles. Educational articles are those that are designed to refresh doctors and often provide great overviews on topics. The *BMJ*, for example, publishes a '10-minute consultation' series and 'masterclass for GPs' series that will provide you with a good overview of the clinical aspects and especially clin-ical skills required for the diagnosis of a condition. Review articles review the published literature and provide an up-to-date summary of the current understanding of a disease, condition or treatment.

The principal free portal to search peer-reviewed journals is **PubMed**, which can be found at www.pubmed.org. It is worth playing with this website early in your studies at medical school, as an advanced understanding of how to use it will benefit you a great deal at all stages of your career. Particularly useful at your stage will be the 'Limits' tab – imagine that you are reading about headache. Putting 'headache' into the PubMed search field will retrieve over 40 000 articles, most of very little interest to you. Now use the 'Limits' tab and put in the following limits:

- articles published in the last year (so up-to-date),
- English language (unless you are multilingual),
- core clinical journals (you are not interested in pure research),
- under 'type of article' click both 'Practice guideline' and 'Review'.

Now hit the 'go' button and you will be offered recent English language articles from the core clinical journals that review the literature or give guidelines for practice. Choose one or two of these and have a read!

If you use information from the article in an essay or your notes, make sure that you **reference** it appropriately, more details about referencing and plagiarism can be found in Chapter 6 and your medical library will be able to give you further information, advice and training. It is worthwhile learning how to reference appropriately as soon as possible, as this is a skill that you will use throughout your career and you can get into hot water if you do not know the rules.

Application examples

Drug names

Many people have trouble learning the names of medications. Antibiotic names seem to be a particular challenge for medical students, so here are some examples of how you could apply the content of this chapter to learning antibiotics.

Cue cards	Have one cue card for each class of antibiotic (e.g. Penicillins), and make a left hand margin for headings, a little like Cornell note taking: • Key examples, • Mode of action, • Bacterial coverage (indications), • Common and serious side effects (SFX), • Interactions and contraindications, • Lesser known facts. Fill a card for each class of antibiotics and carry them with you. In spare moments take a card, cover the right-hand side and see how much you can remember. Repeat as often as needed, initially in order and then after shuffling. Repeat testing yourself again 3 days, 3 weeks and 3 months later.
Mnemonics/songs	Mnemonics are best learnt from writing them yourself and sharing with friends, but here is a useful one from the website www.fastbleep.com

For those of you who like mnemonics, here's a way to remember which are bacteriostatic and which are bactericidal:

We are ECSTaTiC about bacteriostatic

(Erythromycin, Clindamycin, Sulfonamides, Tetratcyclines, Trimethoprim, Chloramphenicol)

Very Finely Proficient At Cell Murder

(Vancomycin, fluoroquinolones, penicillins, aminoglycosides, cephalosporins, metronidazole)

[From www.fastbleep.com/medical-notes/other/21/50/336 permission requested]

Alternatively, if you prefer to hold a tune in your head rather than try and decipher a code:

Try putting 'antibiotic song' into YouTube, or even better, write your own song

Visualisations

Flucloxacillin (Fluclox for short) is one of the few penicillin-based antibiotics that control the bacterium *Staphylococcus aureus*, the bacterium that causes boils, among other things. Imagine a huge flock of clocks flying over a volcanic landscape, except they are not volcanoes, but huge boils, some bursting open, the flying clocks dodging the streams of pus. You will never now forget flew-clocks (fluclox) for treating boils.

Writing mock prescriptions

Download some blank prescription forms from the Internet, start with inpatient forms and make 100% sure that there can be no possible mix up with real forms (write 'for teaching' or something all across each page). Choose a scenario: such as 'a woman with an uncomplicated urinary tract infection', and write up the prescription for what you would like to give her. Check in a national formulary and/or national guidelines whether you got the right medication, dose, frequency and duration. Double check the contraindications and interactions. Finally find one of the online tools for checking that the prescription is legal (date, signature etc.). Note that there are different rules in different countries on what makes a prescription legally valid.

When you get good at this, then start giving yourself more complex scenarios and perhaps getting friends to test you too.

Little black book

Write down every medication that any friends, family, patients that you see are taking, look these medications up – what different uses could they be put to, what interaction would you watch out for if you were prescribing? Many of us are much better at remembering things that we can link to someone we know. Ask your friend/family member to show you the medication, look at it, give it a sniff, ask them if they get any side effects and what the doctor or pharmacist told them about it.

Recycling

In the United Kingdom, the British National Formulary (BNF) is not just a list of medications but also a very decent textbook. Get two out-of-date BNFs (you might have to charm a pharmacist), some sheets of A3 and some glue. At the start of each section is a useful introduction to the type of medications (e.g. Antipsychotics). Glue this in the centre of the sheet of A3. If it goes across both sides of the paper, use the second BNF. Around this central introduction glue one of two examples of each class of medication, like satellites. Use colour, drawings, arrows and keywords to make the sheet more memorable, pin it to your wall and revisit it often.

Posters, Post-its and bathroom tiles

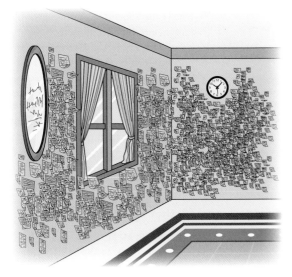

Are you better at remembering locations than lists? If so then you might consider putting a different medication name on each sheet of a Post-it pad (or bits of paper) and stick them in meaningful places around your room (flucloxacillin might go near your clock). Then as you learn about these drugs, write Post-its on side-effects, indications, contraindications, mechanism of action and so on, and stick those around each medication. Look at them often, test yourself and then walk over to the wall and check whether you got it right.

Consider getting a water-soluble felt-tip pen (often called OHP or overhead projector pens, for writing on OHPs back before PowerPoint took over the lecture hall) and use colour and images to write reminders on every tile of your bathroom – how about the mirror where you look every morning. Note that if you have a long bath or shower, condensation will start to act, and you will have to redraw or start another topic.

('Watch out, felt pens stain the grouting between tiles, you might need some grout cleaning solution!')

Peer learning   Start a study group (see Chapter 5) and use it to cover a different class of antibiotics each time you meet. Make sure everyone prepares for the sessions and quizzes each other. Spend some time making sure that you all get the pronunciation correct!

Summary

Learning knowledge is essential for a career in medicine. Learning is an active process that requires effort and engagement. Learning how to learn, just as with any other skill, needs practise (and plenty of it), experimentation and reflection. *Different sorts of knowledge* and *different sources of knowledge* may require different approaches to learning.

References and further reading

Bruning, R. H., Schraw, G. J., Norby, M. M., & Ronning, R. R. (2004). *Cognitive Psychology and Instruction*, 4th edn. Upper Saddle River, NJ, Pearson/Merrill/Prentice Hall.

Buzan, T. (1995). *Use Your Head*. London, BBC.

Cottrell, S. (2003). *The Study Skills Handbook*. Basingstoke, Palgrave MacMillan.

Regarding learning context:

Finn, G. M., Patten, D. & McLachlan, J. C. (2010). The impact of wearing scrubs on contextual learning. *Medical Teacher, 32*(5), 381–384.

Godden, D. R. & Baddeley, A. D. (1975). Context dependant memory in two natural environments: on land and underwater. *British Journal of Psychology, 66,* 325–331.

Questions and answers

Q: How do I know when I know enough?

A: Buried in this chapter are a number of strategies – you can consult curricula, look at the contents of thin undergraduate books, practise past papers, write your own questions (Having read about diabetes, would I be able to explain it to a patient? Let me practise on a friend and see) and, perhaps most importantly, study with others in your year and compare your depth and breadth of understanding with theirs. We discuss more on the pros and cons of collaborative learning in Chapter 5.

Q: What is the point of making notes when I never look at them again?

A: Exactly, you need to build time in to your schedule to review notes regularly. Think about the review when you are writing the notes and plan to make the reviewing as active as possible – perhaps by writing questions or setting tasks that if you can complete will tell you that you know the topic.

Q: My flatmate never does any work and he does really well in his exams

A: Odds are that he studies harder than he admits. Perhaps he just crams for his exams, in which case he will not remember much of what he learnt once the exams are over – do you want him looking after your mother if he qualifies? Why not aim to work harder and become a better doctor. When he fails, he will appreciate your support.

Q: Is this chapter saying that I need to study all the time?

A: Yes and no. You need to be prepared to study over and above the 9 to 5 of the working week. This is the reality of a career as a doctor, and if you just want a 9 to 5 job with great evenings and weekends, you need to take some careers advice. Clearly you need a good balance between study and recreation, and if you are studying all evening every evening, you are doing something wrong. We think that getting the balance right is so important that we have committed a whole chapter (Chapter 8) to the topic.

Q: Writing notes takes ages – would not it be better just to read the book?

A: If you are just starting out making notes, it will take time and effort to improve in speed and accuracy. Think about the words and abbreviations that you use – are you making best use of keywords, headings and drawings? Review your notes – are they too detailed? Have you, perhaps, just copied out chunks of text because it is easier than thinking? Good notes will help you review and revise topics quickly and easily and should guarantee active learning. Your university will run study skills workshops on how to make notes – if you continue to have trouble, why not book into one?

Chapter 3 **Learning clinical skills**

> **OVERVIEW**
>
> This chapter discusses clinical examination and practical skills – how you can work out exactly what you need to learn, how to learn them from books, from simulation and with patients. The clinical learning environment is very different from the classroom environment. We will give you some tips on how to make the most of your tutors and how to make the most of the time when tutors are not around. Finally, we will cover feedback – how to give effective feedback, how to get effective feedback and how to learn from the feedback that you are given.

Introduction

Clinical skills (along with clinical communication skills) are what make doctors. Without the ability to take a history and examine the patient, you will not be able to make a diagnosis. Without practical skills such as cardiopulmonary resuscitation, taking blood and inserting drips, you will not be able to conduct further investigations and treatment. Without effective clinical **communication skills**, you will not be able to explain treatment options to the patient and enable them to understand and to choose the right option for them. You will start to learn these skills at medical school, and you will continue to improve and learn for the rest of your professional life.

The next chapter specifically covers clinical communication skills – the evidence base for learning clinical communication skills, how to make the most from learning in simulation and how to improve your clinical communication skills in the clinical environment. There is a recurring theme in both these chapters, and we make no apologies for highlighting

How to Succeed at Medical School: An Essential Guide to Learning, Second Edition.
Dason Evans and Jo Brown.
© 2015 John Wiley & Sons, Ltd. Published 2015 by John Wiley & Sons, Ltd.

it repeatedly: you cannot learn a skill without knowing how to do that skill, without practising it and practising it a lot, and without receiving feedback. All three parts are important, but practising is the part that is most commonly neglected – compare with any other skill, whether it be playing a violin or playing football – to become an expert, you need thousands of hours of deliberate, reflective practice.

Learning skills is different to learning knowledge, but needs just as much commitment to time and effort. To learn a skill, you need to know how to do that skill (what each step is, why you do each step and what your findings will mean), you need to practise deliberately, thoughtfully and endlessly, and you need to receive and act on plenty of appropriate feedback. If you cover these three aspects, you will be set for life.

To learn anything, of course, you need motivation to learn, appropriate study skills and the self-belief that you can learn whatever the topic or skill is. In this chapter, we will discuss how these aspects relate to learning clinical skills.

On first encounter, the clinical learning environment can be a daunting place. It is unstructured, often chaotic and requires a lot of self-directed learning. If you are seen to be keen and enthusiastic and if you actively seek out learning opportunities, then people will go out of their way to teach you and provide you with even more learning opportunities. You will feel valued and learn lots more than your peers and you will be better prepared for being a junior doctor.

How do I know what to learn?

Finding out the sort of skills that you need to learn at medical school is slightly easier than what knowledge you need to know (Chapter 2); however, the same broad principles apply.

By graduation, you need to have become a safe and competent new (FY1) doctor. This means that you need to be very good at the skills that you will use commonly (taking a history, taking blood, cardiovascular examination etc.) and at the skills that you may need to use less commonly but in an emergency situation (cardiopulmonary resuscitation, or taking an ECG, for example) (Figure 3.1). The next layer down covers the skills that you should be able to do under supervision (perhaps inserting a chest drain or performing a lumbar puncture) – you should have seen and done enough of these to feel confident that you can perform these with a senior watching. Finally, there are skills that you need to know about so that you can explain them to a patient (endoscopy is just one of many examples).

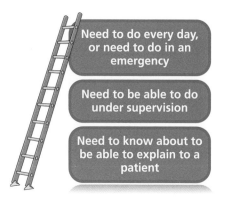

Figure 3.1 Different levels of proficiency are required for different skills.

Your medical school may publish lists of what skills you should gain in a number of formats: this will include being buried in course objectives ("By the end of this workshop on lung function, you should be able to measure a patient's peak expiratory flow rate"), or in year objectives ("By the end of the fourth year, you should be competent at conducting a female genital examination, speculum examination and bimanual vaginal examination and performing a cervical smear") or in your overall curriculum, which may define the skills required for graduation. Many schools publish lists in the form of logbooks or portfolios – for example, at Bart's and the London, we published a 5-year reflective checklist of clinical and communication skills, which showed how skills build on each other year to year, we also had a year-4 logbook, which included clinical skills and a statement in year 5 about skills that might be assessed in the finals.

There are some national publications too. Every few years, the General Medical Council updates 'Tomorrow's doctors', which goes some way to define minimum curriculum content (try www.gmc-uk.org and look under 'education'). Modernising Medical Careers has published a curriculum for FY1 and FY2 (www.mmc.nhs.uk) and other people have had a stab at it too, including the Scottish Doctor Project (www.scottishdoctor.org).

Clinical skills textbooks are not bad either: Macleod's (Munro and Campbell, 2000) and Hutchinson's (Swash and Hutchison, 2002) are two popular ones; a look at the chapter titles gives a reasonable indication of the range of skills that you might be expected to be able to do.

So which list of skills is right? Unfortunately, you are going to have to make some judgements and build a consensus between these different sources. Forget the published lists for a moment and make your own – what skills will you need to be a newly graduated doctor? You might spend an hour or more thinking about this. Structure your list in a way that makes some sense to you (perhaps by body system, or by year of study or by level of complexity). Check some of the other lists available listed earlier and see what you have left out. Keep your list with you, go through it regularly, annotate it and add to it. It will become far more accurate and far more relevant than other people's lists. Perhaps your list could be the first section in your clinical skills folder?

Level of competence

We have alluded to this already: some skills you need to be pretty good at, others you should be able to do with supervision and others you need to

Table 3.1   Benner's model of levels of achievement.

Stage 1: Novice	• Little or no prior experience of the skill • Tendency to focus on the skill itself rather than when to use it or what the results mean • Follow fixed rules that cannot be adapted; this 'rule governed behaviour is extremely limited and inflexible' • Requires full supervision and support
Stage 2: Advanced beginner	• Starts to recognise patterns from prior experience • Starts to use some level of judgement, able to adapt to different situations and contexts • Rules turn into guidelines • Developing dexterity
Stage 3: Competent	• Begins 'to see actions in terms of long-range goals or plans' • Conscious and deliberate planning • Able to adapt to and manage complex contexts
Stage 4: Proficient	• Understands situation as a whole and how one skill fits into complex tasks • Long-term planning: how does this skill, and the way it is performed, affect the future • Appropriate prioritisation • Able to make complex judgements based on experience
Stage 5: Expert	• Accurate, intuitive, unconscious performance • Deep understanding of how a skill fits into the whole situation

Adapted from Benner (1984).
Note that these relate to each skill, an expert at taking blood might be a novice at cardiopulmonary resuscitation.

know about. There are various different grading scales you can use between 'ignorant' and 'expert' (Table 3.1). Clearly, your long-term aim is to become an expert, but at medical school you should aim to become 'good' or at least better than 'good enough' in all the core skills.

Learning clinical skills

A model for the self-directed learning of clinical skills

Learning clinical skills is very different from learning knowledge. The chances are you are pretty good at learning knowledge, with good A-levels and GSCEs. There are plenty of books on improving your study skills for knowledge and Chapter 2 of this book adds to that large body of information. When it comes to learning clinical skills, though, there is very little out there. There are quite a few published papers talking about how the teacher should teach clinical skills, but also plenty of papers telling us that most of the learning of skills that students do is picked up along the way and not formally taught. How best to pick it up along the way is not mentioned.

When looking after students who struggled with clinical skills learning, it became apparent to us that there is often a problem with students not knowing *how* to learn clinical skills. Some students just read the books, without ever practising and then seem surprised when they do not seem to be able to translate knowledge of how to perform a skill from their heads into their hands, to actually perform it. Other students practise and practise, but never get a good idea of how they should be performing a skill. Their clinical skills are often radically different from the norm and they are unable to justify why they do each step. Finally, some students mimic a video or a demonstration and practise until perfect, but without feedback they become very fluent at doing things wrong. In a recent second-year Objective Structured Clinical Examination (OSCE), a number of students had practised using an online video resource for abdominal examination. They said the same words as the doctor in the video and made the same movements, but because the camera angle had not been perfect, they ended up examining mostly the chest rather than the abdomen!

In response to recurrently seeing these problems, we developed a simple model for learning clinical skills (the Evans–Brown model, Figure 3.2). It differs from all the other models in that you, the student, are central to the learning. This is how you will learn as a doctor and this is how most of your clinical skills learning will occur as an undergraduate. The model describes three simple stages – **theory**, **practise** and **feedback**, all overseen by the learner's **frame of mind**.

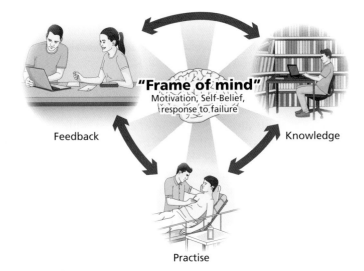

Figure 3.2 The Evans–Brown model for learning clinical skills.

Frame of mind

'I've always been quite clumsy, so I knew that I would have to work harder on my clinical skills to get good'

Rachel, fourth-year medical student.

To learn clinical skills, just as with anything else, you need motivation to learn, appropriate study skills and the self-belief that you can learn the skill.

Just as with learning knowledge, **motivation to learn** is essential and you need a conscious awareness of what motivates you (Chapter 1) and how to manipulate your own motivation if you are going to succeed in learning clinical skills. The concept of '*positive spirals*' is a useful one, actively ensuring that you will feel rewarded for learning, which results in further motivation to learn more:

- Imagine a student is on a half-day placement with the ECG technicians. The technicians ask her if she wants to place the electrodes and run an ECG on a patient. She tells them that she does not know where the electrodes go and they teach her, but she gets a bit confused. Later, when she tries to remember where all the 12 leads of the ECG went, she cannot and decides that it is all too difficult. On her course evaluation, she reports that the placement with the ECG technicians was pointless.

- Imagine now that another student spends 2 hours the night before going to the same placement looking up how to do an ECG, drawing it out on paper and practising (using a pen) on his long suffering flat mate. The technicians ask him if he wants to place the electrodes and run an ECG on a patient. He says yes and gives it a go. The technician is impressed and gives him some feedback on how to improve. During this half day attachment, the student and ECG technician work closely together, and the student does 10 ECGs, really feeling that he is getting the hang of it and even gets some teaching on ECG interpretation. That night he reads more about ECG interpretation and next day he goes in search of ECGs on the ward that he can look at and try to interpret. On his course evaluation, he reports that the placement was excellent and should be compulsory for all students.

The second student was aware that a little bit of preparation would result in reward (praise, obvious learning and feeling good that he could do something), which would then result in an infectious increase in his motivation (*a positive spiral*). In short, he deliberately manipulated himself to become more motivated!

The uncomfortable '**incompetence of learning**' is familiar to many of us. We watch martial arts films or examples of free running/parkour and reckon we could probably do that, but would not dream of trying because, deep down, we know that we would be useless, look foolish and feel stupid. For most of us, that stage when we start learning a new skill, when we are clumsy and completely incompetent, is tough on our egos. Interestingly, some people see this stage as fun, as a necessary and enjoyable part of learning (they see themselves improving rapidly in this stage, which they find rewarding). These people are said to have high **self-efficacy** and they tend to learn much more quickly and effectively. For those of you in the first group, who find those initial stages of learning uncomfortable, you will need to 'grasp that nettle' as early as possible and actively challenge your desire to procrastinate or avoid practising. You might even consider how you could work on improving your self-efficacy. Sometimes learning journals or logs can be helpful to show yourself that you are improving. Moreover, introducing yourself appropriately to the patient as someone who is 'just learning' (see page 57) can be paradoxically empowering – giving you permission not to be competent.

A student's **response to failure** can predict future outcome. Imagine two students fail their third-year OSCE badly. Student A argues that it was not his fault, the exam was unfair, the examiners were not paying attention, there must have been an error in the scanning of the mark sheets and so on. Student B says 'yes, I guess I partied too hard this year and did not do enough work'.

Which of the two students would you be most worried about? There is lots of evidence from **attribution theory** that students who attribute success or failure to factors outside of their control (including being 'too stupid' or 'too clumsy' or 'no good at remembering drug names') do much worse than those with a more *internal locus of control*. If something goes wrong, try writing down what you could have done differently to lead to a different outcome. If it was a particularly painful event, then you might want to wait for a day or two and perhaps get someone to help you think about this aspect (see the section on mentoring, Chapter 12).

EXERCISE

Imagine a student who does not like neurology (low motivation) and feels forced to learn it because it is coming up in the exam (external motivation reduces internal motivation). She has been told by other students and junior doctors that it is a difficult subject, and one tutor told her that she 'probably would not get it' (reducing self-efficacy). She opens a book a couple of times to look at how to do a neurological examination, but she cannot really get into it. She tries to look at a YouTube video but gets distracted looking at cats on the Internet instead. A consultant watches her conduct at a neurological examination on a patient and criticises her heavily in front of a patient. She feels that 'that is so unfair' (negative attribution) and 'I will never get it, this is just too confusing' (negative self-efficacy). Her attendance on the neurology firm drops and she gets away with doing the minimum possible.

Questions

What advice would you give her on:

1 How to improve her intrinsic motivation/interest (perhaps re-read Chapter 1 pages 7–10 [motivation])?
2 How to re-interpret others' pessimism on how difficult it is?
3 How to study effectively?
4 How to improve the feedback that she gets from the consultant, and how to deal with criticism without withdrawing?

How could you apply this advice to yourself?

Building a theoretical framework on how to perform a skill

To perform a skill, you first need to know how to perform it. To play tennis you need to know how to hold the racquet, where to stand in the court, how to strike the ball, forehand and backhand, you need to know the rules, the scoring and 101 other things, otherwise you would just stand there, lost. Similarly for a clinical skill, you need to know how to do that skill – what steps there are to doing it. Imagine that you are going to examine a patient's abdomen – you need some knowledge of what you will be doing before you give it a go.

Often a clinician will show you their way of performing a skill and that might act as an initial framework for you on how to do it. They are likely to tell you that their way is the best way, and it is likely that their way is the best way *for them*, but may not be the best way for you. Have a look in a clinical skills textbook or two to look for other, accepted ways. Have a look perhaps on the Internet and have a look at handouts from clinical skills sessions. They are likely to be similar, but look for the similarities and particularly the differences, try and summarise the steps to perform a skill on one sheet of A4.

> *It used to really bother me that different consultants had different approaches to the same skill, and wanted me to do it their way. It took me ages to realise that over the years I would need to find the way that works for me.*

> Philip, fourth-year medical student.

An interesting model, devised by Martina Michels (2012), identifies three different parts to the knowledge required to perform a clinical skill. The first is the **sensorimotor** aspects, the 'trick' if you like, the steps that you go through: where you put your hands, when. Most clinical skills instructions, textbooks and videos cover these aspects well. The second aspect is an **understanding** of the underlying principles – anatomy, physiology, even basic physics, such as the principles of levers – that justifies why each step is being taken. This is where those students who just watched the video went badly wrong: they just put their hands here or there because that was what was done in the video, they did not *understand* that they were supposed to be feeling for the spleen, or the liver, nor did they know where to find those organs. The final and most complex part of the knowledge is about **clinical reasoning** – making sense of your findings in order to make a diagnosis. Even knowing which examination might be appropriate in which situation.

As an example, let's take respiratory examination. You could be taught the steps of 'how to do it' pretty quickly, and with some practise and feedback, you might get reasonably slick, but you will not understand testing for chest expansion unless you are aware of respiratory physiology and the anatomy of breathing; unless you know the anatomy of the posterior chest wall you will not be aware of the effect that the scapulae have on your percussion and auscultation, if you do not know your surface anatomy, you will not know if you are percussing over liver or lung. And as for clinical reasoning, you need a whole new set of knowledge to help you put together your findings into a diagnosis.

There is a difficulty here in deciding at what level to learn a skill – try and learn too much information (anatomy, physiology, pathology, clinical reasoning *as well as the* 'trick') in one go, and your brain will become overloaded and will forget everything; yet learn just the 'trick' of how to do it, and you might stop thinking and questioning yourself while you examine a patient. If you stop thinking, you will never recognise normal or abnormal.

Our recommendation is that for each skill you have three sheets of A4. We will call these 'skills sheets'. The first sheet contains one side on the 'right way' (your *own* 'right way') of performing a skill (perhaps the steps for a basic knee examination) that you decide on by comparing two or three different expert sources. The second page should contain about one side of the key basic sciences that you need to support the performance of the skill (perhaps the underlying anatomy of the knee joint and surrounding structures). The final page, which you might write only after you have started to master the skill, contains the clinical reasoning – perhaps a heading for each major condition with the key features listed or perhaps a table of key features with their corresponding conditions. This last page is an excellent opportunity for using Cornell notes or tables (Chapter 2).

Practise

Studies of expertise in many different disciplines suggests that about 10 000 hours of reflective, deliberate practise is required to become expert. You cannot get away from this, if you want to become good, you need to practise, practise and practise some more. David Beckham has been playing football 'since he could walk'. The same goes for clinical skills, if you want to be good at taking blood, good at taking a history, good at examining a patient's respiratory system, you not only need to know how to do it, but you need to have done it again and again to transfer that knowledge from your head to your hands.

> *I thought that because I had taken blood pressure once, I knew how to do it. When it came to the exam I was all over the place. I think it takes quite a bit of practice to be able to do things under pressure.*
>
> Ahmed, first-year medical student.

For most skills you would start by practising in **simulation**, perhaps in the skills laboratories, of perhaps on your friends and family. An example of this is that there are two main pulses in the feet that you need to be able to feel – if you can confidently say that they are absent, then that gives a good indication that there is peripheral vascular disease, with a risk of gangrene and amputation, and you can assume that there is likely to be coronary artery disease and cerebrovascular disease too, increasing risk of a heart attack or a stroke. Feeling these pulses is difficult to begin with, but becomes easy with practice. Spend a moment to think about how many friends and family would let you examine their feet; think about how often you sit on the sofa, bored during the television adverts when you could be feeling the pulses in your feet, in those of your flat mates' or your loved-ones'?

Simulation has a role to play in getting you comfortable with a skill and getting over that embarrassing clumsy stage where you are not quite sure what to do next. It is not, however, real and the only way to get good in real situations is by practising in real situations. So when you are competent enough and safe in your clinical skill, go and **practise with patients**. Examining patients is the main way that you will improve when practising your clinical skills for the rest of your life. You might add a fourth piece of paper to your skills sheets, as a log of each time that you have practised each skill, and under which circumstances.

Asking patients for consent to help you learn

Most medical schools now introduce students to patients at an early stage, and a substantial, perhaps the majority of your time studying medicine will be on clinical attachments with patients. We write more about this clinical learning environment later in this chapter. There is plenty written on the ethics of learning with patients and appropriate ways of approaching it, and the BMA does a particularly nice chapter on the subject that should be available in your library and in some institutions as an online textbook (English and Sommerville, 2004). You should have some teaching on how to approach patients and ask for their help in your learning fairly early on in your course. The key things to remember are that the patients need to know who you are and need to willingly give informed consent to help in your learning. The information that they need to enable them to give informed consent includes what will be involved, a true estimate of how long it will take, the fact that it is only for your education and whether they say yes or no will not affect their care and that you have the same duty of confidentiality as other professionals, namely that you will not discuss the patient outside of the clinical team or your learning group. You will be pleased to know that most patients will be eager to help you learn. If the patient prefers that you do not examine them, thank them very politely and then move on to the next patient, they might well feel up to it next time.

Student: Hello, my name is John Smith, I'm a third-year medical student attached to your consultant, Dr Jones. I'm currently learning how to examine the pulses in people's feet and I was wondering if I might examine your feet? It will take no more than 2 minutes and will just involve me touching your feet to try and find where the pulses are – it shouldn't be painful or anything. It's just for my learning, so no problem if you say no.

Obviously, never pressure a patient to allow you to examine them – consent is a gift from the patient and should be given freely. Never allow the patient to misunderstand who you are – if they say 'Yes, of course doctor', for example, correct them 'Oh no, I'm not a doctor yet, I'm a medical student, I'm *just* here to learn'. Not only is this the right and ethical thing to do, but it also stops you from getting into trouble if a patient assumes that you are qualified.

As a basic minimum you must:

- give your name (first and family name) and role;
- explain what you would like to do;
- explain that the interview is for your education only;
- explain that refusal will not affect the patient's treatment in any way;
- explain confidentiality issues, for example, where will this information go; who will see it;
- say how long it is likely to take;
- offer to come back later if the patient is tired, unwell or expecting visitors.

As a student, it is never acceptable to go ahead with an interview, physical examination or procedure if the patient is uncomfortable. Equally though, medical students have a right to learn and many patients value the opportunity to talk to students and contribute to their education. Medical students are often viewed as 'neutral', that is, not part of the medical establishment yet and some patients value the opportunity to talk, particularly as students may have more time than the other health professionals looking after them. Of course, this special relationship may result in a patient telling you something that they have not told the medical team and so it is essential that when talking about confidentiality you make it clear that you may share any information with the rest of the health-care team.

Feedback

Practice on its own is, of course, not good enough. Sportsmen have coaches for good reasons: it is hard to see what you are doing while you are doing it. There are lots of ways of getting feedback: tutors are probably the most obvious candidates, an expert watching you and telling you what was good or bad. There are other ways of getting feedback too: you can ask a colleague to watch you and provide feedback, you can use video or audio taping (but beware that there are all sorts of ethical issues when using this technique with patients, so check these out first) to give yourself feedback and you can ask the patient for feedback ('As I said earlier, I'm a medical student and just learning, can I ask how the questions I asked you about your chest pain compared with how the doctors ask about your chest pain? Did I leave anything out?' etc.).

Not only do you need to receive decent feedback, but you need to act on it too. You can find more information on giving and receiving feedback in Chapter 4. More and more medical schools are introducing portfolios and assessments that require evidence of reflection and action on feedback. You could think about adding to the fourth page (the log) of each skills sheet in your folder with two additional columns on – 'feedback received' and 'action taken'. Not only will this help you to ensure that you respond to feedback, but it will also give you plenty of genuine examples for your portfolio and assessments.

I practised a lot at home on my little brother, but it was only in the retake course that I realised the importance of having other medical students giving me feedback.

Katharine, third-year medical student.

Learning in the clinical learning environment

Transition from secondary school to higher education is a stressful transition, requiring changes to most aspects of your life. There is plenty of research to show that transition from the classroom in higher education to the clinical learning environment (the wards, outpatients, general practice, surgical theatres) is equally, if not more, traumatic. Imagine turning up for your first full day on the wards. There is a timetable with a few sessions on – a ward round here, a clinic there. There are lots of patients. There are few or no tutors visible. There are few, if any, objectives and little supervision. In fact, you could just go home and probably no one would notice. This section aims to give some tips on what to do, how to make the most of what is a pretty unstructured place.

Learning with, from and for patients

There is an increasing move in Medical Education for simulation. 'Simulation' seems exciting, modern, attractive and trendy. Because of this, we can sometimes forget the crux of learning medicine: *Medicine is learnt with, from and for patients.*

Medicine is learnt **with** patients, in partnership. Many patients are remarkably willing to allow students to practice on them to learn to take histories, learn examination skills and learn practical skills. This is a gift that patients give willingly (see the section on informed consent, page 57). You cannot learn to take blood from a rubber arm; you can (and should) *start to learn* in simulation, get over your clumsiness, get used to the different steps of the procedure, develop some degree of fluency, but the only way to get good is to practise a huge amount in reality with genuine, consenting patients (and appropriate supervision etc.). Your task at medical school, then, is to see as many patients as possible.

Medicine is learnt **from** patients. In Chapter 2 (*Learning Knowledge*), we described the importance of context to learning. Things that are learnt in one context are better recalled in that same context. Humans are evolved to tell and hear stories. It is this *narrative* that we hang our learning on. Ask any doctor to tell you the story of their first patient and what they learned from them, and you can expect a story in itself. You will remember medicine far better if you can hang, organise and link those otherwise dry medical facts on to the memories of patients that you have seen. Of course, you learn far more from patients than just information about disease; the patient narrative helps you understand some of the complexities of the person in front of you, in a way that no text book of medicine ever will.

> *Storytelling reveals meaning without committing the error of defining it.*
>
> Hannah Arendt, Social Historian (1906–1975).

Medicine is learnt **for** patients. This might seem like the most ludicrously obvious statement, perhaps patronisingly so, but bear with us for a moment. Bizarrely, patients can be easily forgotten. For medical students, your school's curriculum can and will shift your focus away from patient care and on to the taught curriculum and particularly onto the exams, the exams and the exams. In a rather elegant study in 2009, Ben Wormald (a medical student at the time) and colleagues demonstrated that when the anatomy exams had a low overall weighting that students chose not to study anatomy in so much depth as when the weighting was increased. The fascinating part of their study was that the students fully acknowledged that the anatomy was essential to their work as a doctor and yet still chose not to learn it to the depth that they knew was important, all because it contributed poorly to the end of year score.

Medical students are not the only ones who can easily forget that being a health-care professional is all about providing the best possible care for patients. Every day doctors, nurses, indeed all health-care workers are challenged to forget the primacy of patient care. Whether it be a petty dispute between individuals or professional groups, political power plays within departments or simply as a result of a current political/cultural obsession with judging quality on things that are easy to measure (such as a focus in the UK on patients not waiting more than 4 hours in the emergency department, or a focus on the percentage of staff completing mandatory training, with no consideration for the quality of that training, nor its relevance to patient care).

These challenges are often subtle, almost infectious, within communities. How will you recognise it if your focus has moved away from the primacy of patient care? How will you remedy this shift?

Approach to patients

We have already mentioned consent, but there are some other important issues to consider when learning with patients. Your school will discuss these with you, but as a brief introduction you should be thinking about some of the following issues. Dress is controversial but as a rule of thumb you should be dressed smartly and modestly. In practice, this is likely to mean no trainers, jeans or caps and not showing off your belly (however attractive your piercing is), your cleavage or the top of your bottom (however attractive you think your underwear is). We should not need to mention that you should be clean, groomed (no stubble); you should wear deodorant but not overpowering perfume or aftershave or too much make-up.

You should be aware of infection control, especially how to avoid spreading infections between patients – this sounds easy, but take a look on the wards and count the number of people who do not wash their hands every time, who do not have their sleeves rolled up or who drape their tie or stethoscope over every consecutive patient – make sure that you are not one of them. Short, clean fingernails are essential for both men and women, regardless of fashion or guitar playing careers.

Respect for patients can be demonstrated in a wide range of ways. You should consider your non-verbal communication: looking uninterested, not paying attention or chewing gum will not go down well. The language that you use should reflect your developing professional practice, so think about

Chapter 3

your use of slang terms and street language. You might even ask for feedback on this from your peers and tutors.

Making the most of your tutors

We mentioned earlier on in the chapter that tutors were a good source of feedback, but the truth is that many students are observed very infrequently. Hospitals are bursting at the seams with people to teach you. The only problem is that they usually look busy, flustered and important.

One of our local professors was talking about teaching on the wards and said: 'Those students who just sit around looking bored, I try and avoid them as much as possible, they just get in the way, but those students who are keen and enthusiastic, well, you'll do anything for them, I stay late, I miss dinner, there is nothing better than teaching someone who wants to learn – when I retire I'll really miss them.' One key skill on the wards, then, is learning how to engage your tutors, how to come across as enthusiastic, interested, passionate but not pushy. This is a skill you can learn by watching others and by a bit of trial and error, but here are some tips to start you off.

DON'T

- Turn up late, or with only seconds to spare.
- Sit in the corner of the ward, looking bored – it does not engage others.
- Just wait for teaching to happen – you need to go and find it.
- Sneak off because 'nothing's happening' – if you really, ever believe that there is nothing happening in the hospital that you can learn from, you are in the wrong career.
- Yawn and open a book half way through clinic.
- Assume that only doctors will be useful teachers – nurses are generally better at many practical skills than doctors and have usually been taught how to teach; pharmacists are highly skilled at taking medication histories and in spotting prescribing errors made by the doctors; the physios, the ward clerk, the list of people who you can learn from is huge.
- Assume that only the team that you are attached to are allowed to teach you. Is a psychiatrist visiting your patient? Ask if you can tag along.
- Refuse teaching because 'it's time to go home' – if someone offers to show you something interesting, go for it!

DO

- Look awake and attentive.
- Be early: 10 minutes early should become your new definition of 'being on time'.

- Dress smartly – nothing extreme but smart and modest enough to show that you care about looking 'the part': men should avoid stubble and make sure their shirts are ironed, and women should cover their navel (even if it is bejewelled) and not show their underwear.
- Make the first move: 'I saw Mrs Jones when she came in through casualty, can I watch you do the lumbar puncture?' or 'I was reading about chest X-rays last night, can you tell me what you are looking at on that one?'
- Accept rejection: 'I'm far too busy to teach you right now' should get a reply 'Oh, of course, I'm sorry – is there anything I can do to help, like take forms to X-ray or something?'
- Ask for specific, achievable feedback – asking 'can you watch me while I examine Mrs Patel?' is less likely to get an enthusiastic response than 'can you watch me while I do a 5-minute cardiovascular examination on Mrs Patel, and let me know if you think I'm doing it right?'

Spot the learning opportunities

The last few paragraphs already tried to highlight that hospitals are full of learning opportunities and that students who actively seek them out not only learn more, but also get a reputation for being keen and enthusiastic and so get even more teaching. You can spend any dull moments trying to spot potential learning opportunities and then go out and seize them! The list is endless. We have put a few in Table 3.2 to whet your appetite.

This list in Table 3.2 is not even a start, but will hopefully get you thinking. We have concentrated here on wards and hospitals, but you could equally write lists of opportunities for general practice, operating theatres, outpatient departments and so forth.

As a separate project, one of the authors of this book and an ex-student, now plastic surgeon, asked students, doctors, nurses, patients, physios, chaplains – in fact anyone in or around healthcare – to submit ideas for what students could do when 'bored on the ward'. The little book that resulted from the project (entitled *101 Things to do with Spare Moments on the Ward*) might give you some more ideas; why not get it out of you medical school's library?

How to survive The Business Ward Round

I never learn anything on ward rounds, I'm just the ghost at the back

Leonie, third-year medical student.

Perhaps one of the most controversial aspects of learning in the clinical environment is the 'Business Round'. This is the ward round where the

Table 3.2 Potential learning opportunities.

Drug charts	• Go round the ward looking at everyone's drug charts, look up any drugs you do not know in the BNF (British National Formulary).
	• Ask for a blank drug chart, put a thick line through each page so it cannot be used for a real patient in error and write something like 'medical student practice' under the name. Now write up appropriate drugs for management of asthma, or angina, or heart failure and so on. Ask one of the doctors or the ward pharmacist to comment. Tear it up or take it home when done.
Drug rounds	• The nurses dispense drugs to patients several times a day – why not offer to help: you might get to learn what 'that little heart-shaped pill' that patients keep talking about is and when you sit down to learn about the drugs, you will have heard of most of them before and even be able to pronounce them correctly.
Practical skills	• Patients get their blood pressure, pulse and temperature taken between two and four times a day; on a 20-bed ward that is a lot of practice for you and imagine how pleased the nurses or health-care assistants will be for the help.
Physiotherapy	• Does your patient get wheeled to physio every day? What goes on behind those big swing doors? Why not go and find out?
Radiology	• Read about interpreting radiographs; let us say chest radiographs and then go down to the radiography department and ask what day or time they report chest radiographs; ask if you can come along and watch. The radiologists rarely have students, so you are likely to find one who is keen to teach.
	• Have you ever seen a chest radiograph being taken? How about an abdominal radiograph? Or even an angiogram? What about ultrasounds? All these happen all the time in radiology departments.

medical team, often with other health-care professionals, go round, see the patients, assess their status and discuss options with the patients in order to plan the next steps in their care. It is a fantastic opportunity to learn team-working skills, documentation skills (what do you write in the notes, how much depth etc.), safe decision making, evidence-based practice, professional behaviour, interprofessional working, patient centredness ... the list goes on and on.

Unfortunately, medical students often find these business rounds long and tedious. They feel like 'the ghost at the back', trailing along, wondering if their absence would be noticed if they slipped away. The ward round often progresses rapidly and the discussion is often abbreviated, particularly for patients who have been on the wards for a little while and are known by the team. *'Ah yes, Mrs Gupta. How is her potassium today? … Good. And the CT? Tomorrow? Good. OK Mrs Gupta, I hope we can get you home soon, let's see what the scan shows tomorrow.'* The consultant and the team walk on, the students look increasingly bored. The discussion within the team can be of a higher level than a student can easily understand? – a half explained debate about which high level antibiotic that you have never heard of should be used, which microbiologist to negotiate with and so on. Often there are many patients to see and limited time, so teaching can be conveniently forgotten.

There are two simple options for you as a student – either be bored, switch off and day dream, escape whenever you can or alternatively put your efforts into making sure you learn. Strategies for improving learning include:

- Keep a list of jobs that are allocated to the junior doctors and either volunteer to help during the ward round or just to the junior after the round is over.
- Know two of the patients really well, step forward and say 'Can I present Mrs Jones? I clerked her in casualty last night when she came in with chest pain.' Either they will say yes, or no, they are too busy; however, they are likely to ask you some questions about the patient and to label you as a 'keen' medical student. You can even mention this before the ward round starts and again when you get to Mrs Jones.
- Offer to write in the notes.
- Offer to look up and keep a list of the latest investigation results for all the patients. Step forward in the ward round with Mrs Gupta's latest potassium level.
- Ask questions – 'Sorry, can I ask what potassium level would have you worried?'
- Give up on the factual side and start considering other learning …
  - How does the team interact with the nurses?
  - How well is patient confidentiality maintained? How could this be improved?
  - What communication skills do you see in action between the team and the patient?
  - How about within the team?
  - How are conflicts resolved?
  - Who is leading the ward round? How?
  - There are some published models of how a ward round should run (Royal College of Physicians, Royal College of Nursing, 2012; Herring,

Caldwell, & Jackson, 2011), how well does this ward round measure up? If you were leading the ward round, what would you do differently?

These are just a few ideas that students and staff have come up with, you could easily brainstorm with other students and come up with many more ideas.

Summary

In this chapter, we have highlighted that learning clinical skills is important and takes deliberate, conscious effort. You will need knowledge about the skill, including how it relates to basic science and clinical reasoning, you will need to practise, practise and practise again, and that practise needs to be reflective and linked to effective feedback in order for you to learn. Clinical skills are learnt with, from and for patients; although simulation can help prepare for this, it does not replace the essential role of hands-on practise with patients. Clinical skills (and communication skills) are the fundamental skills of being a doctor – it is worth the investment to make sure you learn them very well indeed.

References and further reading

Benner, P. (1984). *From Novice to Expert: Excellence and Power in Clinical Nursing Practice*. Menlo Park, CA, Addison-Wesley.

English, V., Sommerville, A. & British Medical Association: Ethics Science & Information Division. (2004). *Medical Ethics Today: The BMA's Handbook of Ethics and Law*, 2nd edn. London, BMJ Books.

Evans, D. E. & Patel, N. G. (2012). *101 Things to Do with Spare Moments on the Ward*. Oxford, Wiley-Blackwell.

Herring, R., Caldwell, G. & Jackson, S. (2011). Implementation of a considerative checklist to improve productivity and team working on medical wards rounds. *Clinical Governance*, 16, 129–136.

Michels, M. E., Evans, D. E. & Blok, G. A. (2012). What is a clinical skill? Searching for order in chaos through a modified Delphi process. *Medical Teacher*, 34(8), e573–581.

Munro, J. F. & Campbell, I. W. (2000). *Macleod's Clinical Examination*, 10th edn. Edinburgh, Churchill Livingstone.

Royal College of Physicians, Royal College of Nursing. (2012) *Ward Rounds in Medicine: Principles for Best Practice*. London, RCP. www.rcplondon.ac.uk/resources/ward-rounds-medicine-principles-best-practice (accessed 24 September, 2014).

Swash, M. & Hutchison, R. (2002). *Hutchison's Clinical Methods*, 21st edn. Edinburgh, Saunders.

Wormald, B. W., Schoeman, S., Somasunderam, A. & Penn, M. (2009). Assessment drives learning: an unavoidable truth? *Anatomical Sciences Education.* doi: 10.1002/ase.102.

Questions and answers

Q: Tutors seem too busy to watch me perform a skill.

A: This is a common problem. You do not always need a tutor to watch you, and a colleague might be useful to watch and give you feedback. There are some things that you can do to encourage your tutors – first ensure that you have prepared your skill, so that they do not feel that they are wasting their time teaching you things you could have looked up and second think about limiting the time that it will take. 'Can you watch me take a full history and examine this patient from head to toe – it will take about an hour' is not likely to result in success, but 'I've been practising my cranial nerve examination, I wonder if you might watch a quick 5-minute cranial nerve exam and let me know if I'm doing it right' sounds better.

Q: Every book and every tutor seems to have a different way of examining the breast – which is the right way?

A: The right way of examining a patient's breasts is a method that will be thorough, systematic, will detect pathology and will maintain the patient's dignity and comfort and your professionalism. Check with your medical school; for exams they might expect you to perform a skill *their* way, but for real life, and practice as a doctor, try different acceptable ways of performing skills and work out which is best for you.

Q: Not much seems to be going on and no one checks that I am attending on the wards – would not I be better off going home?

A: You can often get away with only turning up to the timetabled things and slinking off home the rest of the time, but then again, if that is what you want to do, what is the point of you studying medicine?

Chapter 4 **Learning clinical communication skills**

OVERVIEW

This chapter will give you a general introduction to the subject of clinical communication; for example, the professional communication you will be developing as a medical student and as a doctor. We will look at what it is, the reasons for learning it and how to learn it at medical school and in the clinical workplace.

Introduction

'If you can't communicate it doesn't matter what you know'

Kurtz *et al.*, 2005

As a medical student (or prospective medical student), you have already shown that you are good at communicating with others by successfully passing exams, completing a UCAS application and possibly undergoing interviews for medical school or a job. The good news about clinical communication is that it is a subject that can be learned and builds upon the knowledge, skills and views about the world that you already have. Clinical communication *skills* are the physical manifestation of the sum total of your knowledge, attitudes, prejudices and beliefs that manifest themselves when you are working with patients; for example, they are the behaviours that people can observe about you. Clinical communication builds upon your interpersonal skills, which are the general skills you use when communicating with others, such as starting and taking part in a conversation

How to Succeed at Medical School: An Essential Guide to Learning, Second Edition.
Dason Evans and Jo Brown.
© 2015 John Wiley & Sons, Ltd. Published 2015 by John Wiley & Sons, Ltd.

or using and reading body language and so on. Interpersonal skills are important in your communication as a medical student or doctor, and you will be building on these to develop the specialised and sophisticated clinical communication skills you will use as a doctor. So, do not worry too much if communication seems a challenge at the moment, with time and practice, it will become clearer. Clinical communication will become an important part of the clinical toolkit you will develop over the next few years as, during your life as a doctor, you will conduct around 200,000 medical interviews with patients – so it is a pretty important subject (Kurtz *et al.*, 2005)!

Why learn clinical communication?

Clinical communication is the language of medicine and the medium by which medicine is practiced. It is essential in communicating not only with patients but also with colleagues, other members of the health-care team and the wider community. At the heart of clinical communication are the medical interview and the relationship that is built during this between doctor/student and patient. This fundamental relationship is so important and powerful that it can enhance or inhibit the patient's well-being and ability to adhere to treatment and manage their health. Some would argue that this relationship is therapeutic in itself and an essential component of any treatment of a patient. Competent clinical communication is therefore important in providing the best possible care for patients and in enhancing your practice and satisfaction as a clinician. In an interesting study, doctors who were good at communicating with patients and others had better job satisfaction levels (Roter *et al.*, 1997), which seems obvious when you think about it, does it not? Sometimes, students think that the aim of clinical communication is to be 'kind' or 'nice' to patients. This is not the aim at all, as we shall see; rather, think that **effective** use of clinical communication will bring about an empathic, effective and satisfying interview for all concerned. But as well as this, unless you can communicate well, you will be unable to gather a full history from a patient or present that patient's history to a colleague or communicate your thoughts and findings to other members of the health-care team, so effective communication is about being effective as a doctor. We do, of course, also hope that kindness and politeness will always be at the centre of your professional practice as a student and as a doctor, but communication is about so much more.

I thought communication skills classes were a waste of time as I've always been good at talking to people and had lots of experience with my previous job. I found though that they were about something different – proper professional communication. Someone told me clinical language is the equivalent of learning French!

Marcia, first-year graduate student.

Clinical communication is evidence based and it is through extensive research that we know that the physical and psychological health of patients are affected by it and that it plays an important part in most complaints brought against doctors. Did you know that 70% of litigation brought against doctors stems from poor communication (Avery, 1986)? So, clinical communication is constructed from an evidence base that is as scientific as any other part of your clinical course, and in some cases is more so!

When thinking about why we learn clinical communication, it may be helpful to look at some important recommendations made by the General Medical Council as part of the *Tomorrow's Doctors* (GMC, 2011) document, which contains recommendations for undergraduate medical education. The GMC states that medical graduates should:

(a) Communicate clearly, sensitively and effectively with patients, their relatives or other carers and colleagues from the medical and other professions, by listening, sharing and responding.
(b) Communicate clearly, sensitively and effectively with individuals and groups regardless of their age, social, cultural or ethnic backgrounds or their disabilities, including when English is not the patient's first language.
(c) Communicate by spoken, written and electronic methods (including medical records) and be aware of other methods of communication used by patients. The graduate should appreciate the significance of non-verbal communication in the medical consultation.
(d) Communicate appropriately in difficult circumstances, such as when breaking bad news, and when discussing sensitive issues, such as alcohol consumption, smoking or obesity.
(e) Communicate appropriately with difficult or violent patients.
(f) Communicate appropriately with people with mental illness.
(g) Communicate appropriately with vulnerable patients.
(h) Communicate effectively in various roles, for example, as patient advocate, teacher, manager or improvement leader.

Moreover, as part of the Duties of a Doctor registered with the GMC (2013), doctors must

- Treat patients as individuals and respect their dignity.
- Treat patients politely and considerately.

- Respect patients' right to confidentiality.
- Work in partnership with patients.
- Listen to, and respond to, their concerns and preferences.
- Give patients the information they want or need in a way they can understand.
- Respect patients' right to reach decisions with you about their treatment and care.
- Support patients in caring for themselves to improve and maintain their health.
- Work with colleagues in ways that best serve patients' interests.

And so, the GMC supports the learning and importance of clinical communication and the rights of patients to be respected and treated with dignity.

At the beginning of your learning as a medical student, it will be important to think about the kind of doctor you want to become and explore some of the philosophical and ethical positions around this. Developing and exploring humanistic views that value the dignity and worth of all people will provide a good foundation for building views and beliefs about patients and their care, which will directly effect how you will communicate with them. A humanist approach encourages the medical student/doctor to walk alongside the patient, acting as an expert guide but also facilitating the patient to make the best choices for themselves.

> '*I think old school doctors told patients what to do, but nowadays it's all more equal. I feel equal to patients and I'm not some kind of Guru. They have to make decisions for themselves.*'
>
> Aaron, third-year graduate student.

Did you know that during the medical interview, the patient history (the gathering of facts, information, patient ideas, concerns and expectations) by the doctor account for up to 80% of the diagnosis they will come to (Hampton *et al.*, 1975), more than the physical examination or any investigations? So being able to conduct a competent medical interview and gather a patient history are essential to inform clinical reasoning when developing a diagnosis.

Importantly, for you as a medical student, clinical communication forms a core part of the curriculum of all medical schools in the United Kingdom and will be assessed throughout your undergraduate and postgraduate studies. It is as important as any other clinical skill and will demand your time and effort.

Chapter 4

Assessing yourself and others

You probably know quite a lot about general communication already. As a starting point in thinking about your own communication, fill in this communication self-assessment exercise.

EXERCISE

We all need to develop self-appraisal skills if we want to have insight into our own progress and learning needs. Look at the following self-appraisal questionnaire to consider where your strengths and weaknesses lie.

Communication inventory: Think about yourself in this scheme. On a scale from 1 (Low) to 10 (High) rate yourself:

How good are you at listening – really listening?

Do people generally feel comfortable with you?

How good are you at trying to put yourself in someone else's shoes?

How comfortable are you with silence?

How able are you to listen to people's feelings about their problems?

How able are you to listen to people's feelings about their distress?

How able are you to listen to people's feelings about their anger?

How good are you at explaining things to people?

How good are you at recounting events or telling stories?

Could you summarise clearly and accurately something you have just heard or read?

Are you able to tell someone honestly what you think when you know the truth may offend, upset or hurt them?

Are you able to negotiate options when there is disagreement?

(Cushing, 2003)

Now think about these three points:
1 Consider what these answers might tell you about your strengths and weaknesses.
2 How do you know the answers you have given are correct?
3 If you dare, ask someone else that you trust to be honest to fill it out for you and compare what they think of your skills with your self-assessment – what matches and what doesn't?

Now you have a basis for thinking about your own communication and what your strengths and weaknesses are. The important thing is to work on the weaknesses as we would all rather practise the communication we are good at!

Another helpful exercise to spotlight effective communication is to: Think about a personal problem you have had in the past.

- Was it difficult to talk about?
- Who did you talk to about it? (friend, relative, teacher etc.)
- Why did you choose that person, what was it about them that helped you to talk?
- Can you describe the specific behaviours they used?

You may come up with a range of answers such as:

- The person was a good listener, did not interrupt and remembered what you told them.
- You could trust this person not to gossip because you know they are discrete and never repeat private things.
  - The person did not judge you or your actions.
  - The person showed empathy by saying that they could appreciate why you had the problem
- The person was able to give you an honest opinion or advice.

The attitudes and skills that you identify that help you talk about your own problems usually apply to patients who want a doctor who listens well, does not interrupt, remembers the things they say but keeps them confidential, is empathic and is honest and non-judgemental. We can transfer the communication skills that help us directly to our conversations with patients.

My favourite celeb has always been Gordon Ramsay for his straight talking. When I analysed his communication style though I decided he wouldn't make a good doctor!

Shaoib, first-year student.

What are clinical communication skills?

Clinical communication skills cover a wide range of skills but at a basic level concern themselves with:

- eliciting a patient history
- explaining (e.g. a procedure, test, risk or other information)

- exploring (e.g. the ideas, concerns and expectations of the patient)
- discussing informed consent and options
- breaking news
- negotiating (e.g. a management or treatment plan)
- passing on accurate information to colleagues (written or spoken)
  - presenting a case history to colleagues
  - Negotiating a care or treatment package with the health-care team.

As an illustration, let's think about a medical interview and break down the clinical communication skills under rough headings.

A checklist of communication skills

Introduction and orientation	• Welcoming manner
	• Gives name and role
	• Explains purpose of the interview and any note taking
	• Confirms patient's comfort/agreement
Rapport	• Shows interest, respect and concern
	• Appropriate body language (e.g. eye contact, open posture, seating)
	• Matches language and energy levels
Listening skills	• Listens attentively without inappropriately interrupting
	• Responds to patient's answers
	• Picks up on patient's cues (verbal and non-verbal)
Questioning skills	• Appropriate blend of open and closed questions
	• Clear, jargon-free questions
	• Clarifies when necessary
	• Avoids leading questions
	• Keeps note taking appropriate
Empathic responses	• Reflecting back and acknowledging patients' feelings and concerns as expressed in the interview

Information giving and explaining	• Checks what patient knows/understands • Gives clear jargon-free explanations • Well paced (chunks and checks) • Invites questions, checks patient's understanding • Draws/uses diagrams where appropriate
Respecting autonomy, negotiating and shared decision-making	• Proposes options, their benefits and risks and helps the patient make their own decision • Refrains from judgement, threats or irritation
Appropriate reassurance	• Handles uncertainty appropriately • Refrains from false or premature reassurance • Offers appropriate reassurance or help
Closure	• Summarises main points to ensure everything is covered and information has been gathered accurately • If applicable, explain next step
Organisation of the interview	• Summarising • Signposting • Systematic and logical flow

(Cushing & Brown, 2001)

This checklist shows the main **process** headings of a medical interview and breaks these down into skills. The **content** of the interview is the information that is gathered or given, driven by the knowledge and attitude of the doctor or student. So we may say that some clinical communication skills are the **process** skills that enable the **content** to be gathered – essentially you cannot have one without the other!

The next diagram called 'The Patient Centred Clinical Interview' (Levenstein *et al.*, 1989) gives us a model of the medical interview that illustrates a fundamental underpinning principle of effective clinical communication, that of 'patient centredness' (Figure 4.1). This term is used in the model to describe the 'illness framework', which is the framework used by the doctor to explore the ideas, concerns and expectations of the patient in order to understand them. The model shows that the doctor has two

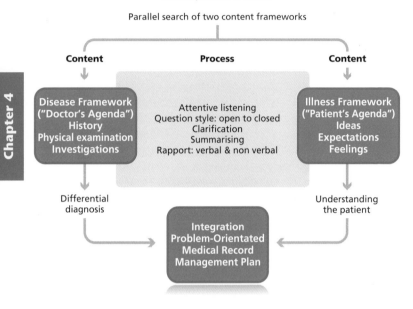

Figure 4.1 Patient-centred clinical interview.

tasks in the medical interview, to understand the patient and to understand the disease, and that through exploration of these parallel frameworks an informed and patient centred diagnosis can be reached.

The thing to know about good clinical communication skills is that they help to build the **relationship** between the student/doctor and the patient. Without this, any medical encounter will be poor and lacking in satisfaction for both parties.

Thinking about empathy

An important part of building any kind of relationship, and one of the underpinning principles of communicating with patients that you will learn as a medical student, is the important topic of **empathy**. There are many definitions of empathy but it is essentially about your ability to walk a mile in the patient's shoes, or to appreciate, understand and accept someone else's emotional situation (Cohen-Cole & Bird, 2000). Empathy is different from sympathy, which is about feeling sorry for someone. But can we really feel empathy for every patient all of the time? Students often worry about this and, of course, the answer is, not always! There are two ways of categorizing empathy that you may find helpful.

Affective empathy (Cox *et al.*, 2012) – or feeling empathy. As you might have guessed, this is where you *feel* empathy for someone, you are able to create a similar emotional state to them just by observing them. We all experience genuine affective empathy for some patients which can be triggered by all sorts of things, for example, they may remind us of someone who is close or they present with a situation that we feel is genuinely distressing or unfair. You will experience affective empathy with many patients, but not all.

Cognitive empathy (Cox *et al.*, 2012) – or thinking empathically. This is where you are able to take on board and accept someone else's emotional state or situation by focusing and thinking about it, but you do not necessarily *feel* the empathy. Cognitive empathy should form part of your practice and is important in day to day practice where the situation is less emotionally based or intense or when you are dealing with more everyday events.

Cognitive empathy plays an important part in patient centred practice as it can be used authentically in any encounter, even when we dislike someone or when we are having a difficult day (Spatz, 2013).

So, it may be helpful to have a definition of clinical empathy to work towards, which is the ability to:

- Understand and appreciate the patient's situation, perspective and feelings,
- Communicate that understanding and check its accuracy,
- Act on that understanding with the patient in a helpful and therapeutic way.

Adapted from Mercer and Reynolds (2002).

Pause for thought

Firstly, think about a medical interview you have experienced personally (GP visit, occupational health, outpatient clinic etc.) using the definition above, was the doctor empathic? If so, what kind of empathy were they using do you think? If not, would it have been helpful to you if they had?

Next, think of a person that you find difficult to like. It might be that you dislike their appearance, or the things they say or the way they say it. Or maybe you do not agree with their world views? Using the aforementioned cognitive and clinical empathy definitions, would you be able to treat them empathically in a clinical situation?

Chapter 4

Exploring and trying to genuinely understand what is going on in a patient's life provides a greater depth of understanding of their situation, builds a strong relationship and aids diagnosis and treatment.

How are clinical communication skills learned?

You are already reading about clinical communication and this is a good place to start. At the end of this chapter are some references for books that will help you look further at some of the theories and models of communication if you are interested. However, clinical communication cannot be learned entirely from books and must be learned by **practising or doing them**. This is sometimes called **experiential learning** and may be different from some of the learning you have done in the past. Experiential learning encourages you to actively try things out in a practical way and learn from the results. It encourages you to build upon the experience you already have and use this as a basis for developing new knowledge and skills. Think about this next activity as an example.

Chapter 4 *(margin tab)*

EXERCISE

An Example of Experiential Learning

In order to practise your information-gathering skills, you decide to interview a friend about his recent trip to the GP surgery for a sore throat.

You talk to him for about half an hour, asking questions and gathering details of his story. You might write some of this down in order to practise taking notes.

At the end of the interview, you ask your friend for some feedback about how the interview went and how he thinks you did.

He tells you that you made him feel comfortable at the start of the interview by looking interested in what he was saying. He says that you were very clear that the reason for the interview was for you to practise gathering information and that you asked clear and straightforward questions. He also explains that he would have liked to tell you how frustrating it was to wait 45 minutes to see the GP and how apprehensive he felt when the GP took a throat swab, which actually made him want to vomit, but he did not feel that he could interrupt your flow of questions and as you were looking down to take notes he couldn't catch your eye to interrupt.

On the way home you think about and reflect on the interview. You realise that you were successful in gathering information from your friend but that you got so carried away with asking him your questions and taking notes that you did not give him an opportunity to tell you about the things that were important for him. You decide that next time you interview someone, you will start by asking them to tell their story first, before asking your questions and so start with what is most important for them.

Moreover, you decide to spend less time looking down at your notes and more time maintaining eye contact to pick up body language cues.

Using role play to learn clinical communication skills

Many medical schools use role play as part of experiential learning. Role play allows you to try out or practise a patient interview in a simulated setting (a classroom or group learning room) with a simulated patient (an actor, another student or sometimes a specially trained patient). A role play group should be thought of as a safe laboratory for experimenting where any explosions will be harmless! And so do not be afraid to try things out, experiment and see what works best for you as this is a golden opportunity and there is no such thing as a perfect role play. We all have different ways of learning and some people may feel less comfortable about learning with role play, but just resolve to give it a go, jump in at the deep end and see how it feels. Many people who feel apprehensive at the start go on to really enjoy and value role play as an effective way of learning clinical communication. In fact, all the research tells us that experiential learning and role play are the best ways to learn clinical communication initially and that it is important to practise these skills as much as possible. As we have already mentioned, it takes 10, 000 hours of deliberate, reflective practice to become an expert and at least 100 hours until you become reasonably competent at a skill (Anderson, 1982; Bruning *et al.*, 2004). Clinical communication is no different and so practise, practise, practise makes perfect!

The usual set-up is for a role play session to be carried out in a small group with a tutor. There is usually a predetermined patient scenario that has been written to allow particular skills in a relevant clinical situation to be practised. In its simplest form, each student tries out a role with an actor or simulated patient for a short time and then gets feedback on their performance from others in the group. Sometimes there is an opportunity to re-do parts of a role play to see if things turn out differently and sometimes the role play can be filmed to allow the role player to see themselves in a particular situation. Seeing yourself on film can be a nerve-racking experience the first time, but students rate this highly as a very useful learning experience. You often have to watch the film several times until you get over seeing and hearing yourself on screen and can look at what is actually happening in the role play. There is a practice role play at the end of this section if you would like to try it out.

Chapter 4

Feedback

Feedback is an essential part of role play; in fact, you cannot have one without the other. We all need feedback from others to get a different perspective on our performance and just as we saw in the experiential learning example, often we are not aware of some of our own behaviours and how others may see or be affected by these. Giving and receiving feedback should be an honest and constructive experience. Feedback is not about character assassination or comments of a personal nature, but should be focused on a person's **behaviour** in a given situation, helping them to develop new perspectives or behaviours if appropriate.

An example of this may be that you have watched a fellow student talking to a patient and noticed that the patient was finding it difficult to hear because the student was speaking so softly. The feedback you may want to give would be centred on the student speaking louder and also watching the patient to pick up cues that they found it difficult to hear; this feedback would allow the student to think about their behaviour next time and possibly change it. What you would *not* give feedback on is the student's voice itself, which is personal, probably cannot be changed and will result in them feeling hurt or personally criticised.

Behaviours and skills are not in themselves 'good' or 'bad' – it depends on the effect they have and if they are achieving the objectives. When giving someone feedback, remind yourself to look at what worked well at the same time as what might be improved and consider suggestions for how to improve things. This is important for a reason other than kindness, as at any given moment we can only put a certain amount of energy towards changing ourselves. It is a help to know what we already do that works well and therefore does not need to be looked at. We can then concentrate more easily on other suggestions for change.

Some Feedback Tips
- Whenever possible allow the person whose skills are being evaluated to do a self-critique first. Usually, people in this position are very critical and find it difficult to describe what they have done well. Although they may need to deal with any problem they experienced, it is also important to point out aspects that worked well.
- When you give feedback, you may find that all you have to do is emphasise points already made by the person whose skills are being discussed. If not, make two or three comments, but always by describing (behaviourally) what

you saw, why you think it is not the best way (refer to the effect it had on the patient) and what you suggest would be an improvement. Try to make it a habit to write down some of your comments so that the person can read them later.

- Always focus on what you see by describing behaviours. For example, rather than saying something general like 'You're doing OK', try something specific like 'I liked the way you checked to make sure Mrs Jones understood your explanation'.
- There is a difference between the intention behind our behaviours and the effect they have. For example, rather than say 'You made that patient embarrassed' (which may not have been the intention), try something like 'When you …, I thought the patient looked embarrassed'.
- Remember that **all feedback is subjective** and the person receiving it may disagree.

(Cushing, 2000)

Chapter 4

So, it is important to be specific about behaviours when giving feedback. Concentrate on a particular part of an interview, and give examples and perhaps write down some of the words that are said – this will aid your memory and act as a reminder for the person receiving the feedback. It is also important not to overwhelm people with lots of feedback that they probably will not remember! Try to limit feedback to the **three most important things** you saw.

When I saw myself on DVD doing a role play I couldn't believe how awful I looked and sounded – I had to go over it with friends lots of times. Eventually I could see what I was doing and it was really helpful to have that perspective.

Phoebe, third-year student.

Feedback can be a tricky skill to get right and needs practise: we all enjoy giving positive feedback but find negative feedback more difficult. Interestingly, students say that they value honest feedback from colleagues and teachers above all else and find it the most helpful way to learn. Working in small groups with colleagues allows you to develop an honest and trusting group relationship that fosters constructive and honest feedback.

Giving and receiving feedback will be important skills to develop over your medical training as they will not just be needed for role play but for a range of things throughout the rest of your professional life. Someone who regularly gives and receives feedback will be in tune with others and not just relying on their own thoughts and opinions.

You might like to practice a roleplay with colleagues including giving and receiving some constructive feedback. Here is a roleplay to start you off:

EXERCISE

A practise role play

You may like to practise a role play with two other colleagues. Person one should play themselves as a medical student, person two should play the patient, and person three should time the role play (say, 5 minutes) and give feedback to person one.

The instructions for **person one** (the medical student) are:

You are on your General Practice attachment. Mr/s Smith has come in today with stomach pains and has agreed to see you before she/he goes in to see the GP. Please introduce yourself and take a focused history of what has brought them in today.

Person three should apply some of the principles from the feedback section and using the 'Communication checklist' on page 74 – should give some feedback.

The roleplay for **person two** to perform is:

Epigastric pain roleplay

Background details

Your name is Joe/Josephine Smith and you are a 31-year-old restaurant manager. You have lived locally all your life. You work long hours, maybe 60 per week, mostly working evenings and weekends. You are passionate about food and really enjoy your job and the contact with the customers and restaurant staff. You know you are good at what you do and you earn a high wage. The restaurant owner is appreciative and supportive of you and you have worked there for 3 years. You are divorced, live in a one-bedroomed flat close to the restaurant and do not tend to have many friends as your social life revolves around the restaurant. You do not have any children and you do not have a partner at the moment, in fact your relationships do not tend to last very long.

Lifestyle (occupation and effects on life, smoking, drinking, diet, exercise and leisure)

The restaurant can get pretty stressful at times and you like to blow off steam at the end of a shift by drinking wine with the senior chef. You often drink a full bottle of wine each evening and two or three times a week will follow this with a couple of large whiskeys to help you sleep. You do not drink alcohol at any other time of the day. You smoke 20 cigarettes a day and take no exercise as you feel your active job is enough. You are on your feet for long hours and keep on the move. On your day off, you tend to just sleep and watch TV as you are exhausted. You do not bother with breakfast and eat lunch and dinner in the restaurant – beautiful, rich food. You are very partial to beef in all its cooked forms. You weigh 80 kilograms.

Presenting problem and history (Why you are here today and what has lead up to this, any ideas about what the problem is or concerns about the problem, what do you want from this consultation?)

You have a pain in your stomach, which is getting increasingly worse. This last three days, it has made you miserable and it has been almost impossible to work through. It is a gnawing pain in the centre of your stomach that seems to run back into your spine. It now wakes you at night and you cannot sleep through it. It first started 5 months ago and you noticed it occasionally, but it was mild. Now it is there most of the time and seems to get worse when you eat food. For the last couple of days, you have eaten very little but have been drinking to dull the pain. You have tried Rennie and the chemist suggested you to take Zantac, which worked at the beginning, but now does not touch it. You have noticed that your stools are quite dark and smelly – you are embarrassed about this. You do not like doctors but were forced by the pain to come today. Your mother is alive aged 54 and is well. She suffers with mild arthritis but is very active. You do not have any siblings and are not aware of any other stomach problems in your family.

Ideas, concerns, expectations (private thoughts, fears, mood)

You know you drink and smoke too much but do not want to be lectured by the doctor. You will be cagey about how much you drink unless the student is non-judgemental. If you suspect any judgement, you will be deliberately vague. If you feel listened to and the student seems sympathetic then you will be more forthcoming. Your dark fear is that you have stomach cancer as this killed your father when he was 40 – very near your own age. You just want this pain to stop so that you can get on with your job. Normally you are a very affable person and people comment on your hosting skills in the restaurant. You fear being told to give up smoking and drinking or being advised to take time off. If treated empathically and you feel respected by the student you will answer questions honestly – you are not stupid and know

things have to change. If you feel judged, you will close down and just keep
returning to the stomach pain.

**Make sure that you all rotate through the roles, so that everyone in
the group gets a chance at playing the patient, playing themselves
as well as giving feedback**

You get the idea of role play from this. You can write role plays yourself
using this model about any clinical area or situation to practise with peers.
Clinical communication skills are the only skills in medicine that continue
to get better as you practise them – they never reach a peak, but continue to
evolve and develop as you use them throughout your clinical career.

Giving information

We have looked a lot in this section at the communication needed to gather
information, but some of the most complicated communication situations
doctors face are those that involve giving information to patients or colleagues. We know quite a lot about how we retain and recall information
from research carried out about memory, but how often do we really think
about how information is received, understood and remembered? We know
from research that we remember best when we are relaxed and calm and
do not feel that we are being tested in any way! We also remember the first
and last things we are told fairly well, but may not recall some things in the
middle. We also remember things best when they are broken up into logical
chunks and we are able to have a conversation around them to really explore
and understand them – this principle is how we learn most things really. It is
also important to check someone's understanding of what we have told them
to ensure that we have been clear and our information has been understood.
Just asking someone 'have you understood?' is not enough as politeness and
pride forces us to say that we have, even when this is not true!

Table 4.1 may be a helpful guide.

**It is important to know that you will never be called upon to give unsu-
pervised information to a patient while you are a student,** but it is good
practice to observe and critique those around you who are doing it. You could
try out the following role play, with a peer playing the patient, to practise your
information giving skills. Or even better, you could try it out in a group of
three to allow for feedback:

EXERCISE

Medical student information

You are on placement with the respiratory team and are attending the respiratory clinic today. The consultant has asked you to speak to Kasia/Pavel Zak who attended today for review of her/his asthma. She has suggested that Mr/s Zak has a flu vaccination but as the clinic is running late, has asked that you explain the following information to the patient. She will return to answer any questions later in the clinic.

Flu information to explain to the patient

Flu is a highly infectious and common viral illness that is spread through coughs and sneezes. It is not the same as the common cold as it is caused by a different group of viruses. Symptoms are more severe than a cold and last for longer. You can catch flu all year round but it is more common in winter and it cannot be treated with antibiotics.

Symptoms include high temperature, headache, general aches and pains, tiredness and sore throat. You may feel nauseous and develop a cough.

Flu can be more serious for people with long-term conditions such as asthma as it can exacerbate the symptoms and it is therefore recommended that asthmatics have a flu vaccination to prevent it.

A flu vaccination does not give you flu as the vaccine contains inactivated flu viruses. You may experience a sore arm near the injection site and some people may get a slight temperature and aching muscles for a few days afterwards. Other reactions are very rare, but you should not have flu vaccination if you have had a reaction to it in the past or if you are allergic to eggs.

People need an annual flu vaccination to combat the different strains that emerge each year. The vaccine is available from October each year through the GP Surgery.

Kasia/Pavel Zac roleplay instructions

You are 23-years-old and have had asthma since you were 7. Your asthma is well controlled with inhalers and is only really a problem if you get a cold or exercise too rigourously. You have been in the United Kingdom for 2 years since coming from Poland and have recently started a new job in a shop. You have heard of flu vaccination before in Poland, but are not convinced about having it as some of your friends developed very bad flu after having the vaccination. So, you are a bit uncertain about having the vaccination, but if the medical student explains it to you clearly you will probably agree. You do not think you are entitled to sick pay in your new job so certainly do not want to get ill with flu.

Table 4.1   Model on information giving.

Preparation	Think about what you are going to say, gather together any facts or diagrams and think about 'how' you are going to say things
Context	Explain the purpose or context of the information. When beginning, signpost your agenda 'Can we talk about three things today'?
Check	What does the patient know already? What is their starting point? How much information would they like or need today?
Check	Throughout the meeting check what they are feeling and thinking about – this allows them time to process the information and you the opportunity to check for any misunderstandings
Chunk	Give small, logically linked chunks of information for patients to process
Conversation	The meeting should be a conversation that allows both parties to contribute to and take part in. Questions may come up at any time
Language	Calibrate this to the patient. Check their level of understanding of English language and check whether they can hear you clearly. Make sure you share the same understanding of terms. Avoid or explain medical jargon
Pace	Check whether you are going too fast
Check understanding	Ask the person to tell you in their own words what they have understood or remembered 'Just to check that I have explained that clearly, I wonder if you can tell me what you have understood'?
Cue recall	Remind them of the topics you agreed to discuss and orientate them to each as you discuss them
Other forms of communication	Use drawings, diagrams, graphs, online websites and leaflets to explain

Adapted from St George's, University of London (2013).

How easy was it to give this information? Were you able to use the Information Giving model to guide you? Next time you see someone giving information, critique what you see and decide how you are going to do it in future. There may be opportunities for you to give information to patients under the supervision of a qualified doctor – seek out these opportunities.

Learning clinical communication skills in the clinical environment

At some point in your course, you will begin to learn and take part in the clinical workplaces of hospital wards, outpatient clinics and general practice and primary care. For some people, this will be the most exciting and rewarding part of their course and for others it may seem quite unstructured and therefore a little daunting. The work you may have done experientially will be a good preparation and foundation for this part of the course where you will be talking to and learning from real patients.

The clinical environment offers wonderful learning opportunities, but sometimes it is difficult to recognise them, particularly if you are the kind of person who likes very structured activities with a tutor taking the lead. We remember our own experiences of going on to a ward for the first time and not knowing where to physically 'be' for most of the time. Everyone seemed to be very busy, very confident and knew what they were doing: it took a few weeks to settle in and find our places in this new world. Everyone feels like this! The vital thing is to realise that you have to make learning opportunities for yourself as clinicians will have competing priorities and will not be able to offer support all the time. It may be helpful to plan your day around the structures that already exist, such as ward rounds, surgeries and clinics.

Ask yourself:

- How can I prepare for the upcoming ward round/surgery/clinic?
- Which patients should I be talking to and examining today?
- How will I get feedback on what I am doing today?
- How will I record what I have learned today?
- Which other members of the health-care team should I be working with today?
- Can I help with any jobs, for example, taking a sample to the laboratory?

At this point, it is important to mention informed consent and patient rights. You will remember that these were covered more fully in the clinical skills chapter.

In the clinical workplace, you will be introduced to 'clerking', which is taking a full history and performing a full examination of a patient. At first, this will take quite a while and you will need lots of practice. Aim to fully clerk five patients per week and this will soon add up to a substantial number – remember each skill takes 100 hours of practise in order to achieve a minimal competency. By interviewing patients regularly, you will learn how to approach them and build rapport, how to find out about their story and record this accurately, how to elicit their concerns and fears and find out about their health beliefs and how to examine them competently.

The more you talk to patients and immerse yourself in the clinical environment the easier things will become. If you are the kind of person who finds it difficult to approach a patient or strike up a conversation, try to prepare for this in advance by **visualising** what you will do.

Chapter 4

- Visualise yourself walking over to the patient.
- Visualise how you will greet them – what words will you use?
- How will you go through the steps of informed consent – what words will you use?
- Will you ask for permission to sit down?
- What opening line will you start off with – the weather, their journey, photos on the locker, asking about lunch?

This technique is useful for preparing yourself. It may also be helpful to jot down the areas you would like to talk to them about on your pad to act as an *aide-memoire*. A simple history template is sometimes helpful:

- the presenting problem(s)
- history of the presenting problem(s)
- past medical history
- family history
- medication history
- social history
- review of systems

A tip here is not to prepare the questions you are going to ask but simply to be curious about your patient and their story and really listen to what they tell you. Remember that the medical 'history' is simply 'His Story' in a more structured way. Often students stop listening and miss information because they are concentrating on the next question they are going to ask. Listening is one of the most important clinical communication skills. You also should avoid asking 'checklist' questions guided by the history template – patients' do not tell their story according to a checklist. Your job is to **map their story** onto a clinical template rather than the other way round.

This is a good point to introduce you to a model for gathering a patient history. This model (Figure 4.2) is an adapted version of the *Calgary Cambridge Guide* (Kurtz *et al.*, 2005), which breaks the medical interview down into five steps: initiating the session, gathering information, the physical examination, explanation and planning and closing the session. At the same time, it provides two pillars that run through the five steps and outline the skills that provide structure for the interview and build the relationship with the patient. You may want to use this as a template for your interviews with patients.

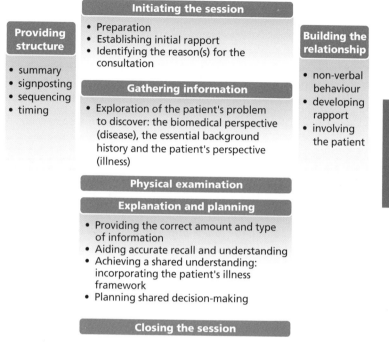

Figure 4.2 The Calgary Cambridge Guide: a guide to the medical interview.

The Calgary Cambridge Guide will provide you with a foundation for gathering a patient history and you may like to experiment with it to see how it fits in with your particular interviewing style.

Where possible and appropriate, try to interview patients in pairs initially. This allows one of you to talk to the patient while the other observes and gives feedback. If you are feeling really brave you could also ask the patient to give you some feedback. Remember that feedback is the key to good clinical communication and that the more you receive, the better and more skilled you become. Try to get feedback from a variety of people so that you get a wide perspective on your skills. It will be important to ask qualified doctors and nurses to watch you for a few minutes with a patient and then give you feedback. You may like to ask them for specific feedback; for example, supposing you have identified that you have a tendency to interrupt patients before they have finished telling you something or that you find it difficult to use open questions when taking a patient history, ask for specific feedback about these, it can be really helpful to pinpoint specific things. But you must also bear in mind that *all* feedback is subjective and opinion-based, which is why gathering a variety of views helps to maintain a balance.

> *One of my interviews in the third year was with a patient who cried when we talked about his wife who had recently died. I felt useless at the time, but the next day when I went back he said he was comforted by me just listening to him and thought I would make a good doctor*

Muna, fourth-year student.

Not all interviews with patients need be long or very formal. In some settings such as outpatient clinics or GP surgeries, it may only be possible to speak to patients for a short time. Gathering and grabbing all opportunities to talk to patients is the vital thing and will help you build up an extensive and varied experience base. A useful tip is to keep a patient interview diary (ensuring that you do not use patient names or identifiers), where you write down the various interviews you conduct, what were the strengths and weaknesses, what you have learned from these, and what to try out next. It may also be helpful to record the particular types of histories or examinations you have done to make sure that you have a wide experience; for example, if you have spent some time interviewing patients about their respiratory problems, perhaps you should aim to do the same with patients who have diabetes or are about to undergo a procedure or operation of some kind? This way you have a clinical log as well as a reflective journal of clinical communication.

Thinking about diversity

Have you ever stopped to think about the sort of person that becomes a medical student in the UK? Do you think of medical students as being a homogenous group? If you had asked these questions 50 years ago, the answers might well have been 'yes, medical students tend to be middle class, privately educated, male and white'. Of course, in the increasingly globalised world we live in today, the people who become medical students have changed in line with the rest of society. Women, for example, now make up 55% of the medical student population with a prediction that this figure will increase to 65% in the future (Lempp & Seale, 2006). White men now make up just 26% of medical student numbers and in some medical schools students from ethnic minority backgrounds make up nearly 40% of the population (Lempp & Seale, 2006), with an increased number of international students encouraged to study medicine at UK universities. These crude figures only give us a glimpse of the people who become medical students of course and give us no clue as to other issues about them like socio/economic background, religion and world beliefs, sexuality, political persuasion, health experiences and beliefs and so on. But, although we all know intellectually that society has changed in the UK and is now made up of a rich diversity of people, with a rich diversity of lifestyles and beliefs, and although we believe that we embrace this diversity and these differences, do we really?

> '*Patients mostly think I am a nurse because I am female, I always have to explain that I am not*'

Cindy second-year medical student.

Stereotyping

A working definition of stereotyping is the knowledge that we hold, and the assumptions that we make, about groups of people and the characteristics that we perceive they share. Psychologists believe that we stereotype as a way of learning about the world by sorting and grouping things from an early age, for example, children stereotype tigers as being generally dangerous even when the tigers look different from one another (Moskowitz *et al.*, 2012). In other words, we sort individuals into groups that we perceive have particular qualities or behaviours as a quick way of understanding them.

EXERCISE

Pause for thought

Do people stereotype you as a medical student? What characteristics do they believe you share with other medical students? Are some of them true? Are some of them false?

In medicine, we also link some diseases to certain population groups, for example, hypertension is common in south Asian populations, sickle cell disease affects Afro-Caribbean and some Mediterranean populations, Ashkenazi Jews have a higher prevalence of Tay Sachs disease and so on. So we are taught to categorise some patients according to their social or ethnic groups in order that we may sort them into appropriate health domains (Moskowitz *et al.*, 2012). Studies have shown that this is a helpful way of developing useful health information about a patient, but that as well as dealing with this biological information, we may trigger inaccurate beliefs in our mind about the behaviour or characteristics of these groups that are negative. You probably know about the way beliefs are built – you see a woman driving poorly and so you ascribe all women as poor drivers, you read about a crime committed by a man from a specific ethnic group and you ascribe all members of that group with criminal activity (Rhodes *et al.*, 2012) – we all do it, but studies suggest that we stereotype people, mostly unconsciously, and that most of us deny we do this because we are simply not aware of it! (Moskowitz *et al.*, 2012). In an interesting American study that looked at the unconscious stereotypes that hospital doctors held, they found that these stereotypes negatively influenced the diagnosis and treatment decisions that they made about black and white patients (Green *et al.*, 2007). So, we need to be aware that we can be influenced by our own unconscious need to stereotype people and that this may influence the way we make decisions about or treat patients. We need to develop an awareness of our thoughts and attitudes and how these might affect others.

EXERCISE

Think about the following scenario for a few minutes:

You are on a GP placement and have been asked to talk to Lauren Peters, who is a 20-year-old woman with a history of drug and alcohol problems. Her clothes are scruffy and she appears to be quite anxious and uptight. She has two young children with her who look dirty and uncared for.

Lauren tells you that she has lost her prescription for painkillers for her bad back and also that she has come to request that her coil is removed because she and her new partner want to try for a baby. She will see the GP in a few minutes.

Now ask yourself some questions:

How does she make you feel?

What issues does this situation raise?

What information might you want to gather about her?

What stereotypes might affect this patient?

Some issues that might arise for you

Maybe you have been thinking about whether women with drug and alcohol problems should be allowed to have children? Does this scenario raise any child protection issues? Should the children be taken away from her? Perhaps you are worried about her having a new baby? Has she really lost her prescription?

What kinds of questions are you going to ask her to explore all these areas?

Thinking about stereotyping; what are the real issues here, her drug and alcohol problems or perhaps her poverty? Lots of people are long-term heroin or methadone users and we simply just do not know who they are, is she more visible because she is scruffy and the children are dirty? Think about someone like the famous model Kate Moss – she is a very successful model who allegedly used cocaine while she had a small child. What differences are there between her and Lauren Peters, which somehow makes her alleged drug problems more socially acceptable?

(Turner, 2013)

What we have to learn to do is treat people as individuals no matter what stereotypes they may fall into as there is as much variation within groups as there is between them. It would be impossible in such a diverse world to try to learn about all the various cultures that exist and, anyway, we know that patients do not conform to stereotypes. The key to establishing individuality is to really ask people about themselves and their needs and beliefs. As a society, we are often reluctant to do this as it feels risky or maybe asking someone about their ethnicity or sexuality feels too sensitive or politically incorrect – but how else can we find out about their individuality unless we explore it? By really finding out about a patient, we also test and challenge our stereotypes instead of leaving them in splendid isolation to secretly influence our perceptions and decisions – we become culturally curious and in tune.

EXERCISE

Think about this next patient:

Mrs Jennifer Onyeador is a 74-year-old Nigerian woman who lives alone in a small flat. Blood tests reveal that she has poorly controlled type 2 diabetes for which she is prescribed Metformin tablets. She has come to the diabetic clinic today as she has a leg ulcer that will not heal properly.

What would you want to talk to Mrs Onyeador about? What would be important to explore to ensure that you treat her as an individual? What are the issues? Think about the questions you would ask her to find out about her lifestyle, diet, habits, finances, housing, exercise, family, hobbies, smoking, drinking, recreational drug habits, health beliefs and background?

Only when you have explored all of these will you have a complete picture of her life and can then begin to think about how her diabetes is affecting this.

So, think about the following three things when you are next with a patient: Have you got a stereotype in your head?

What is influencing your thoughts or actions?

What questions are you going to ask to find out about this patient?

Chapter 4

Chapter 4

Presenting patients

Learning how to present a patient and their case history in the clinical work-place is an important area of clinical communication that brings together your clinical knowledge, ethical thinking, history taking and examination skills with clinical reasoning. You make this presentation as a way of telling those assembled what is known about a particular patient, what investigations and examinations have been done and what differential diagnoses (e.g. hypotheses) you have arrived at. It is a time honoured way of co-constructing clinical thinking and diagnosis with a range of colleagues to share thoughts and reasoning. Presenting a patient is an excellent way to learn as it helps you to put together and prepare what you know in a systematic, logical and clear way that facilitates clinical reasoning. You will usually be invited to present the patient by a senior doctor in front of a range of others, including the patient themselves, which can be a tricky situation to manage.

Presenting in this way to colleagues is often called Case Presentation and different types of these exist:

- **Bullet presentations** (very fast, 1 or 2 minutes in length) are usually given during a ward round, in a corridor or over the telephone. It is a very quick description to introduce a patient to a new audience, for example:

  '*Mr Rahman is a 45-year-old secondary school teacher who presents with knee problems for three months and was found for the first time to be hypertensive. As an enthusiastic runner, Mr Rahman is anxious to have his knee problem resolved*'.

- A **formal Case Presentation** (around 5–7 minutes in length) is usually given to supervisors and colleagues at the bedside or in a sit down conference.
- A **complete Case Presentation** (around 10 minutes or longer in length) will outline the full medical details about a patient. Junior doctors are expected to make these as part of the Foundation Programme.

(Joekes, 2012)

You will notice that each presentation is for a different **purpose** and that purpose is determined by the **context** of the presentation. To introduce the team quickly to a patient, you would use one method, but to thoroughly go over all known clinical details you would use another. Similarly, you can imagine that the **type** of information will be contextually driven also. Different information will be needed for a patient at different stages of their health-care journey; for example, what might be important information to know about someone when they are brought into the Accident and Emergency Department by ambulance will be very different to that needed a week later when the team are planning the discharge of the patient.

So what topics are included in a case presentation? The following might be a useful guide:

- An outline of the diagnosis (if known) and its presentation in the patient.
- An outline of clinical reasoning (how the diagnosis was confirmed, for example, history, clinical tests etc.).
- Treatment including pharmacological, surgical and any other interventions.
- Recovery (response to treatment, psychological and physiological).
- Discharge plan (the ability of the patient to manage once discharged).
- Notable points that may include features of the patient's past medical history, occupation, social history or unique life experience and so on.

Moreover, you will notice that these topics are dependent on the stage of the patient health-care journey and are context specific.

This may seem a little daunting to you at the moment and certainly learning how to present a patient is a complex skill that will take a lot of practise. But you will get better as you progress through your course and gain experience. Each senior team will also have a preferred method for presenting patients so it will be important to find out what this is and to prepare for it.

So what clinical communication skills might be helpful in a case presentation?

Have a look through this list:

- Introduce yourself and your patient
- State the purpose of the presentation (e.g. assessing treatment, planning for discharge, unusual medical problem etc.)
- Present the information in a structured and logical way (with flexibility to allow for questions)
- Emphasise notable points
- Give specific information
- Summarise key points
- Say if there are any outstanding issues or points about which you would like guidance
- Make a clear closing statement
- Exclude jargon

(Joekes, 2012)

All this is done at the same time as managing the relationship with the patient! This can be a complex thing to do, so imagine yourself in the patient's shoes for a minute in the next exercise:

> **EXERCISE**
>
> You are (make up a name) sitting on a surgical ward having had your fractured leg pinned surgically following a bike accident. You are 2 days post surgery and still in some pain, which is controlled by medication. You are worried that the leg will not heal well enough to allow you to run the half marathon you had planned for later in the year. In fact, you vaguely remember someone saying that you would need physiotherapy for some weeks after the plaster comes off. Just after breakfast the consultant and all the other doctors and nurses gather around your bed and one of the medical students starts telling them about your bike accident. **How could the medical student involve you in the conversation and make you feel included?**

So, however complex presenting a patient must seem at the moment, you must resolve to practise it many times. Grab any opportunities you have on the ward or in clinic and at the end of any history you gather from a patient, think about how you would present it to senior colleagues.

Summary

In this chapter, we have looked at the definition of clinical communication, why it is used and how it can be developed and practised in a simulated setting. We have thought about the diverse world we live in and have looked at ways of applying clinical communication skills in a clinical environment with real patients and with clinical colleagues and at the importance of feedback for learning and development. We have looked also at the doctor/student–patient relationship and the importance of empathy to this.

- Clinical communication is not about being 'kind' or 'nice' to patients.
- Good clinical communication is essential to clinical competence.
- Clinical communication is evidence based.
- Listening and curiosity are key communication skills.
- Empathic communication underpins the doctor/patient relationship.
- Practise and feedback are essential to the development of competent clinical communication.

References and further reading

Anderson, J. R. (1982). Acquisition of cognitive skill. *Psychological Review*, 89, 369–406.

Avery, J. K. (1986). Lawyers tell what turns some patients litiginous. *Medical Malpractice Review*, 2, 35–37.

Bruning, R. H., Schraw, G. J., Norby, M. M. & Ronning, R. R. (2004). *Cognitive Psychology and Instruction*, 4th edn. Upper Saddle River, N.J., Pearson/Merrill/Prentice Hall.

Cohen-Cole, S. A. & Bird, J. (2000). *The Medical Interview: The Three-Function Approach*, 2nd edn. St Louis, MO, Mosby.

Cox, C. L., Uddin, L. Q., Di Martino, A., Castellanos, F. X., Milham, M. P. *et al.* (2012). The balance between feeling and knowing: affective and cognitive empathy are reflected in the brain's intrinsic dynamics. *Social Cognitive and Affective Neuroscience*, 7, 727–737.

Cushing, A. M. (2000). *Guidelines on Giving Feedback*. London, Barts and the London School of Medicine and Dentistry.

Cushing, A. M. (2003). *A Communication Skills Self-Assessment Form*. London, Barts and the London School of Medicine and Dentistry.

Cushing, A. M & Brown, J. (2001). *Communication Skills Feedback Form*. London, Barts and the London School of Medicine and Dentistry, p. 1.

GMC. (1995). *Duties of a Doctor: Guidance from the General Medical Council*. London, General Medical Council.

GMC (2011). *Tomorrow's Doctors. Outcomes and Standards for Undergraduate Medical Education*. London, General Medical Council.

GMC (2013). *Good Medical Practice*, Manchester, General Medical Council.

Green, A. R., Carney, D. R., Pallin, D. J., Ngo, L. H., Raymond, K. L. *et al.* (2007). Implicit bias among physicians and its prediction of thrombolysis decisions for black and white patients. *Journal of General Internal Medicine*, 22, 1231–1238.

Hampton, J. R., Harrison, M. J., Mitchell, J. R., Prichard, J. S. & Seymour, C. (1975). Relative contributions of history-taking, physical examination, and laboratory investigation to diagnosis and management of medical outpatients. *British Medical Journal*, 2, 486–489.

Joekes, K. (2012). *Tips for Presenting to Colleagues*, student handout, St George's University of London.

Kurtz, S. M., Silverman, J. D. & Draper, J. (2005). *Teaching and Learning Communication Skills in Medicine*, Oxford, Radcliffe Medical.

Lempp, H. & Seale, C. (2006). Medical students' perceptions in relation to ethnicity and gender: a qualitative study. *BMC Medical Education*, 6, 17.

Levenstein, J. H., Belle Brown, J., Weston, W. W., Stewart, M., McCracken, E. C. *et al.* (1989). Patient-centred clinical interviewing. In: Stewart, M. & Roter, D. (eds) *Communicating with Medical Patients*. Newbury Park, CA, Sage Publications Inc.

Mercer, S. W. & Reynolds, W. J. (2002). Empathy and quality of care. *British Journal of General Practice*, 52 Suppl, S9–12.

Moskowitz, G. B., Stone, J. & Childs, A. (2012). Implicit stereotyping and medical decisions: unconscious stereotype activation in practitioners' thoughts about African Americans. *American Journal of Public Health*, *102*, 996–1001.

Rhodes, M., Leslie, S.-J. & Tworek, C. (2012). Cultural transmission of social essentialism. *American Journal of Public Health*, *109*, 13526–13531.

Roter, D., Stewart, M., Putnam, M., Mack Lipkin, J., Stiles, W. *et al.* (1997). Communication patterns of primary care physicians. *JAMA*, *277*, 350–356.

Silverman, J. D., Kurtz, S. M., Draper, J. & Kurtz, S. M. T. (2005). *Skills for Communicating with Patients*, 2nd edn., Oxford, Radcliffe Pub.

Spatz, A. (2013). *Empathy Workshop*. St George's, University of London, London.

St George's, University of London (2013). *Information Giving, Principles and Practice Workshop*. Undergraduate MBBS Education.

Turner, M. (2013). *Stereotyping – A Workshop for Undergraduate Medical Students*. London, St George's, University of London.

Questions and answers

Q: I find it difficult to disturb patients to talk to them as I cannot help with their treatment.

A: It is quite true that talking to patients is for the purpose of helping your learning and education, but patients quite often enjoy talking to students and may feel this is a way of practically helping with your education. It is also true that you have a right to be a learner and that although the needs of the patient must be uppermost, the best way for you to learn is by talking and practising.

Q: I find the wards quite bewildering. I never know which patients to talk to, or whether it is OK for me to talk to them?

A: Everyone feels like this at the beginning. The important thing is to agree with your clinical supervisor which patients you will approach as he/she will be able to guide you and may want you to look at specific patients, perhaps because there is a ward round coming up or because the patient is about to return home and so on. The vital thing is to treat the clinical environment as a place of learning and try to gain as much experience as possible.

Q: A patient that I particularly got on with told me something she had not told the doctor.

A: This sometimes happens, which is why it is important that when you obtain consent to interview a patient that you explain you cannot guarantee confidentiality between you, but that any information will be shared within the health-care team. Importantly though it will *not* be shared *outside* the health-care team, which includes the patient's family, friends or workplace and so on. You will need to discuss any additional information you gather about a patient with their supervising clinician.

Q: It takes me a long time to take a patient history, sometimes over an hour. Nobody else seems to take this long.

A: At the beginning, it is common to take a long time to interview a patient. Over time, you will become more comfortable with the process and more proficient at interviewing or examining a patient. Enjoy this time and make the most of being with patients in an unpressured time frame.

Q: Sometimes it feels like I am prying into the patient's private life when I take a history.

A: This is a common and understandable concern but there is a clinical *reason* for asking a patient personal questions. In the normal run of things, a patient would not dream of sharing such information with you, but as a medical student you are in a privileged position in which you are able to ask patients in-depth questions about their lives. You seek out this information in order to take a full and competent clinical history, it is not done as part of curiosity or prying but as a clinical skill.

Chapter 4

Chapter 5 **Working in a group**

> **OVERVIEW**
>
> This chapter gives you some useful tips on how to build and maintain produc-
> tive group work. Group work is important in medicine both as an undergradu-
> ate and as a doctor, so we hope that this chapter will help act as a springboard
> for effective team working and team learning for many years to come.

Introduction

As a medical student and as a doctor, for the rest of your professional life you
will be required to study and work with others. We have already highlighted
the importance of working in a study group, but we have not given you much
guidance on how to get one together, how to make it work. This chapter will
help you identify your personal preferences when it comes to group work
and will describe some of the pros and cons. We will dip into some practical
theory from educational psychology to consider why and how things can go
wrong and what the key strategies are for making it go right.

The second half of this chapter will focus on the specific challenges of
problem-based learning (PBL) groups, self-study groups and interprofessional learning. You will also find useful advice relevant to study groups for
clinical skills in Chapter 3 and clinical communication skills in Chapter 4.

What do you think?

Different people have very different perspectives on learning in a group. Some
love it, some hate it. This perspective is partly due to some level of inbuilt preference (whether from nature or nurture, some people tend to be 'loners'), but

How to Succeed at Medical School: An Essential Guide to Learning, Second Edition.
Dason Evans and Jo Brown.
© 2015 John Wiley & Sons, Ltd. Published 2015 by John Wiley & Sons, Ltd.

it is largely due to past experience. Consider the exercise you did in Chapter 1, p. 12. How did you answer the question on group work?

EXERCISE

Think back to a typical example of group work from your past, try to recall the session in your mind or even in writing. Ask yourself the following questions:
- What was the task?
  - In what way did the nature of the task affect how the group worked together?
- What about the make-up of the group?
- What were the behaviours between people in the group?
  - Which were helpful?
  - Which were unhelpful?
  - Were any behaviours particularly destructive?
  - What did the group do about these?

Spend another couple of minutes thinking about the following question:
- What would be the characteristics of a task that encouraged productive group work?
- What would be the perfect list of different characters or personalities or skills in the group for productive collaboration? You might want, for example, someone who is good at finding information, someone else who is good at motivating the group. What others can you think of?

Your prior experience is important; if you have had positive experiences in the past, then you are likely to be the sort of person who will engage positively with future experiences. The opposite is true too. This is important to be aware of – other members of the group might behave in ways that help or hinder the group's productivity, but so do you. Go back to the earlier questions and consider what behaviours that you had in the group and what effect it had.

Some friends invited me to join their study group for clinical skills. We set a topic in advance, but I didn't really prepare. They ended up teaching me and one of them got quite angry that they were only covering the basics, and I got angry back. I never went back, which is a shame – it's hard to learn clinical skills on your own.

Colum, first-year medical student.

Pros and cons
There are, of course, pros and cons to working in a group. Some are real, others are more subjective. Some are fixed, whereas others can be influenced in

ways that we will discuss later. We do not plan to produce an exhaustive list here, and we are sure that you could add more, but we will try and provide a balanced list (Tables 5.1 and 5.2).

Of course, working in a group is not all roses, and you have probably come across some difficulties and disadvantages; we list some typical problematic situations in Table 5.2.

Table 5.1   Advantages of working in a group.

Collective knowledge is more than individual knowledge	You will never know everything, others will always know things that you do not know and you will always know things that others do not know. You can always learn from others
Collective skills are more than individual skills	As you will see later, different people tend to have different roles within a group. You may not be as good at finding information as one of your peers, but perhaps you are better at spotting links across topics or getting an overview or 'helicopter view' of the topic. Together you are stronger than apart
Learning through teaching	One of the best ways of checking that you understand something is by explaining it to someone else; if you can do this, and answer their questions, it will consolidate the facts in your head much more deeply
Depth and breadth	We have mentioned the problem of depth and breadth quite a lot. Throughout your time at medical school, you will struggle with knowing when you know enough. The three main ways of telling are through exam results (too late), by looking at the learning objectives (often not specific enough) and by measuring yourself against your peers (by working in a group)
Hidden curriculum	For good or for bad, the grapevine carries a lot of information about the curriculum. Students who work alone are often unaware of things that everyone else knows. ('I just didn't know what to expect for the exam' when every other student in the school knew what the questions were last year and the year before)
Motivation and empathy	We all have bad days. Days that we do not seem to be able to get round to doing work, that nothing seems to make sense. If someone you trust tells you that they had a similar experience last week, then you might decide to give it another go tomorrow. Perhaps they also struggled with the same topic and found a really useful way of looking at it that will help you too
Divide and conquer	For some tasks (not all tasks), many hands really can make light work, especially if you coordinate your efforts well. Often tasks can be divided up between you and then recombined to make a good finished product far more quickly and easily than it would take one person alone

Table 5.2   Disadvantages of working in a group.

You know a lot more than them	When you know a lot more than the rest of the group on a topic, then you can spend a disproportionate amount of time explaining very basic things when you could be using that time more productively alone
You know a lot less than the rest	If most people in the group seem to know a lot more about the topic than you, the level of discussion can be so high that you have trouble following. You might just sit there, listening to a foreign language and get frustrated at the waste of time or demoralised at your lack of knowledge
Disorder and disharmony	We have all worked in groups where people tended to shout each other down a lot, play one-upmanship and try and win points over the others. Often this is a normal stage that a group can go through (Table 5.4), but sometimes the group can be stuck in chaos and struggle to be productive
Individual behaviours	Sometimes one or two individuals can have behaviours that make it difficult for the group to function. Perhaps they get angry or put others down. They often do not realise, but sometimes they do
Not sharing the workload	Colum's quote highlights a relatively common phenomenon when some members of a group do not 'carry their weight'. If they never or rarely prepare, they become seen as 'hangers on' and resentment can start to build in the group

The difficult truth

Love them or hate them, the clean and simple truth is that you will need to learn to work in a group. At medical school, you will benefit from doing some of your study in a group (you cannot learn clinical or communication skills without it, for example) and for the rest of your professional life you will be working in teams.

The people in these teams will not always be people who you would choose for friends, but you will need to learn to value them for their strengths and recognise and support their areas of weakness, and they should do the same for you. Similarly, in study groups, you may not always work with people who are your friends, but you can still be amazingly productive.

We hope that we have convinced you that you will need to work in groups, that there are advantages and that it is not always plain sailing. The rest of this chapter looks at how you might help the group to be as productive as possible.

Roles within a group

Back in the 1980s, Dr Raymond Meredith Belbin published his investigation of management teams in industry. His work identified that for a team to work

Table 5.3 Belbin's model of team roles.

Chairman/ coordinator	This role involves coordinating the others, delegating the right jobs to the right people and providing focus on the task
Shaper/motivator	Shapers tend to be full of enthusiasm and motivation for the task. They are keen to 'win' and their passion overflows to others. They can be quite aggressive in their aim to achieve
Plant	These are bright, intellectual lateral thinkers. They are great at coming up with ideas, different ways of doing things
Monitor/evaluator	People in this role are those who keep an eye on deadlines and progression towards them. They will think things through and propose the most sensible path. Often they are pragmatic and may be a little cynical
Company worker	This is the role that gets the work done; they are loyal to the team and get the work done on time
Team worker	This role is interested in building the team spirit and keeping everything running smoothly. They are the diplomats and tend not to take sides
Completer/finisher	This role is interesting. It involves producing a suitable finished product – dotting the 'i's and crossing the 't's, checking the spelling. Ironically, their high standards can frustrate others and actually lead to delays in completion (so not, perhaps, the best name)
Resource investigator	This role involves actively seeking out sources of information, external contacts and building networks outside of the team

Adapted from Watkins and Gibson-Sweet (1997).

productively people took on different roles within the team, with some people taking on more than one role. He came up with some rather strange names for the different roles, which we will try and summarise here (Table 5.3). As you read through them, see if you can identify with them from teams that you have worked or studied in.

The interesting thing about Belbin's model is that not only can one person play more than one role within a team, but also people may play different roles in different teams. Moreover, people tend to have roles that they are good at and roles that they find more difficult. Imagine that you are a perfectionist who prefers to do things right. You will probably be comfortable putting things together into a final product (completer/finisher) and might be quite reasonable at many of the other roles too, but you will find it more difficult to delegate and so might find it harder work to fill a coordinator role.

This Belbin model is not perfect and our brief description of it is rather superficial, but it does give a framework with which to look at a group that you are working in and consider some of the reasons that there might be challenges.

Imagine the following scenario: four of you have been selected to produce a poster on health in the local community.

- If none of you take on the role of resource investigator, then how will you find the data that you need?
- If no one takes on a coordinator role, then how will you avoid everyone doing the same things?
- If everyone takes on a coordinator role, how will you ever agree on what needs to be done?
- If no one in the group has attention to keep the team together, then who will ease things over when you cannot agree on a background colour for the poster?

The Belbin roles allow you to do more than just understand why things are going wrong. You can actively use this framework to ensure that the group becomes productive

- You might consciously decide to invite people to join the group who you think will fill in the gaps – if you do not have an obsessive-compulsive proofreading completer/finisher in the group, and your posters tend to look rather tatty, perhaps you could invite one to join you, regardless of whether you like their company or not.
- You might use the Belbin framework to have a discussion in your group – perhaps you are all keen to lead and none to follow, if you can talk about this, perhaps you could rotate the role of coordinator.
- You might also use the framework to personally think how you will work within the group. You are likely to be pretty good at four or more of the roles and probably reasonably good at another two or so. Imagine that no one in your group is very good at keeping the team spirit up and you know that with some effort you can do that, you might decide to throw yourself into that role, even though it is not your strongest preference.

Watkins and Gibson-Sweet's article (1997) is a good starting point if you wish to read more. They even give a different analogy of teamwork, useful for those who find Belbin's roles too abstract.

Group dynamic, group development

Groups do not start functioning at 100% capacity straight away. They often go through a rocky period in the first few meetings. You know this from experience and Bruce Tuckman formally described it in 1965. He described four stages that a group goes through before they start 'performing' (Table 5.4).

Table 5.4 Bruce Tuckman's four stages of team development.

Forming	At this stage, members of the group are polite and try to understand each other and the unwritten rules within the group. They avoid conflict and their comments tend to be generic or ambiguous so as not to risk disagreement
Storming	The politeness ends here and the conflict begins. This might be conflict about the right way of pursuing the task or vying for leadership or respect within the group. Members are more willing to disagree and conflict may range from members talking each other down all the way to displays of anger
Norming	In this stage, the group has learnt the unspoken rules of how they will work together and they develop trust and respect and become a true team
Performing	Having successfully navigated the previous three stages, the group become truly productive

Adapted from Westberg and Jason (1996).

The strange thing about the model in Table 5.4 is that it appears to be true. Almost all groups seem to go through these stages, although some get stuck at one stage or another.

The relevance to you is twofold. First, if on the second or third time your group meets, people seem to stop getting on, perhaps they start talking each other down and argue a bit, then you can be reassured that this tends to happen and most groups will move on to start performing within a couple more meetings. In addition you might think about how you might help a 'storming' group to move on to a more productive stage. Your group tutor (if you have one) should also help, but your role within the group will put you in a position of influence. Consider what you have read about feedback (Chapter 4) and reflection (Chapter 7) and use this to provide feedback for the group and stimulate them to think about the processes going on. Examples might include the following:

- *'I notice that we tend to keep interrupting each other a lot, and we seem to lose out on a lot of information by not listening, could we think about some ground rules for the group?'*
- *'We seemed to be getting along so well last week, I wonder what was different between then and now.'*

Other factors affecting learning in a group

There is a lot of evidence from educational psychology that various factors other than development of group dynamic and roles within a group also influence the productivity of the group. In this section, we will list them, give brief descriptions and some practical suggestions.

Products/goals

Goals that are more concrete tend to produce more interaction (although unfortunately also less breadth of learning), so you might wish to help your group make its goals as concrete as possible.

- 'So to summarise, when we meet next Thursday we will all be able to list all the causes of clubbing and we will construct a table of what other clinical features would point us to each of those diagnoses.'
  Goals that are shared between members of the group tend to be better than goals that are divided up between individuals. Although the goals should be shared, individuals should still be accountable within the group.
- You might start a session going round members of the group to find out how they prepared for the session. Often this is in the form of people talking about what sources of information they found.
  The nature of the task itself seems important, with tasks that require everyone's input having a better effect on group interaction. Concept maps, for example, seem to be better than a poster or an essay that one person could make on their own.
- Work hard to ensure that everyone has input to the final product.

Individual factors and positive interdependence

Although prior knowledge is important, for a group to learn and grow effectively together they should have a similar level of prior knowledge. We hinted at this when talking about the cons of group work. Although the members of the group do not need the same prior knowledge, clearly if one person is an expert and the others are novices the session will become simply a teaching session, at the cost of group motivation and the importance of debate, discussion and elaboration.

- Try to ensure a similar level of prior knowledge – encourage members to do the study that they agreed before the session and discourage those who try to read ahead of everyone else.

'Positive interdependence' is a term used to describe that everyone in the group should require the others to complete the task or to complete the task well. Groups that appreciate that their results are better because of the different members of the group tend to continue to perform well.

- Try and ensure that the goals are owned by everyone (as above).
- Help the group to consider the strengths of its members – perhaps you could say something positive about everyone's contribution.

Chapter 5

Behaviour within the group

If you read Chapter 2, you will not be surprised that **asking questions** (especially questions that encourage deep understanding), elaboration and trying to build links with other learning will result in deeper learning and better group performance.

Ask questions, be curious, try and apply the knowledge that you are sharing and try and link with other learning. Ensure that you are all actively learning in the group.

> *Someone in my group kept asking 'why' and we really found it irritating to begin with, she persevered and suddenly we realised that we couldn't really explain the things we were saying, we didn't understand as deeply as we had thought. We were quite shocked and had to go back to the books. I now think that 'why' is one of the most powerful questions.*
>
> Jason, third-year graduate entrants' programme student.

Whereas emotional conflict can be quite destructive in a group, **cognitive conflict** can help ensure deep learning and a common understanding. Cognitive conflict refers to a disagreement on a thinking, rather than an emotional, level and it tends to stimulate motivation, curiosity and reflection.

- Ask questions that will stimulate curiosity and challenge fixed views, such as: 'If, as we read, a fasting blood glucose of ≥ 7.0 mmol/L diagnoses diabetes, but why 7.0 rather than 6.9 or 7.2?'

> *'I love a good debate, and so did the others in my group, we learnt a lot by disagreeing with each other.'*
>
> Abdul, final-year medical student.

Interestingly, the more that the interaction in the group is **structured**, the better the learning outcomes tend to be (but at the cost of free thought). This might well be part of the advantages of some of the highly structured models of collaborative learning such as PBL, but it can also work to your advantage in less formal settings.

- Consider setting some ground rules for how the group wants to work. Perhaps for revision sessions, you will agree to always start with a brainstorming session on the topic, followed by a review of the learning objectives set by the school, and you follow that up with making up some questions individually and trying to write model answers for them as a group. You will find these sessions much more productive than just turning up to 'revise diabetes'.

Understanding **other people's point of view** is one of the most important parts of working in a group. We talked about empathy with patients in the chapter on clinical communication and empathy with others in your study group is just as important. Often emotional conflicts occur because individuals are more interested in pushing their own point of view rather than truly trying to build a consensus. For a consensus to form, everyone needs to see each other's perspective and try and see how it relates to each of the other members' perspective.

- If you find that the conversation keeps jumping – student A makes point X, student B makes point Y, which is unrelated to point X and student C interrupts to make a different point – then try proposing this simple exercise: whenever anyone speaks, they summarise what the last person said and build on it. Give it a try, it is harder than it sounds!
- If different opinions are flying wildly around the group, consider stepping out of your own opinions and into a facilitative role. For example:

> 'This is interesting, we seem to have three different opinions here. If I can just summarise where I think we are at, Jacob seems to argue heavily that prostitution should be legalised so that it can be regulated, but Malini thinks that this will just encourage an explosion in an already crime-ridden area. It seems to me that there was also a second debate, more focused on the women themselves, with Peter keen that they become destigmatised and supported, and I think the only way that he saw this happening was through legalisation. Could we agree that this summary is broadly what we have covered so far? OK, so should we brainstorm what we know about regulation, association with crime and stigmatisation in prostitution?'

You will not be surprised to hear that just as with individual learning, group learning is driven by **motivation.** Some are motivated externally (we have to work together to get this assignment done) whereas others are driven by interest in the topic, or the feeling of unity with the group or by the interactions and cognitive conflicts within the group (Abdul's quote earlier, for example). If you can maximise this motivation, in yourself and others, the group is more likely to be productive.

- Consider talking about what motivates you and starting a discussion. If everyone knows that you are interested especially in the pure science and another group member is more motivated by relevance to patient care, then you can make sure that your discussions are tailored for both of you.

Chapter 5

Special cases

Problem-based learning

PBL is simply a structured way of going about group work. There is some evidence that students who learn in this way are more highly motivated and learn more deeply, integrating their knowledge together more effectively. As a result of this, there are plenty of medical schools where the vast majority of the information that students learn is learnt through PBL, your school might be one of them. Medical educationalists are passionate about PBL (they either love it or hate it) and, it probably goes without saying, there are lots of different flavours of PBL, with their different proponents arguing that theirs is 'the' right way. Some schools use the term case-based learning (CBL) to refer to the sort of learning that we are talking about here, but others use CBL to mean something rather different.

The PBL group is made up of students (including a chairperson and a scribe) and a tutor. There are perhaps six to eight students in a group, sometimes more, and one takes the role of chairperson. This 'chair' keeps order, guides the group through the steps of PBL and ensures that everyone has their say. A different student takes the role of scribe – writing things up on a board, usually a whiteboard, and capturing the discussion. The scribe has quite a position of power, and of responsibility, as they can direct how things go by the way that they write things down. Innovative scribes, who use colours, concept maps and flow diagrams, tend to drive innovation in the group. Scribes who just tend to write lists can sometimes have a very negative effect on the group. The most remarkable thing about PBL is the role of the tutor. The tutor does not teach. He or she should act as a facilitator only, keeping in the background, supporting the chair and scribe, occasionally asking a question or nudging the topic gently one way or another and sometimes challenging unhelpful group behaviours.

The learning in the group centres on a problem and a structured way of thinking about that problem. The problem itself is usually something relevant to the topic and often relates to a realistic context. Good problems should stimulate curiosity and motivation and make the students puzzled, keen to find a solution. Good problems should be difficult or even impossible to 'solve' – the learning comes in thinking and debating and reading and testing hypotheses, not in finding the 'right' answer.

We stated that there were different flavours of PBL, here we will run through the seven-jump process that is used in many medical schools in the UK. It came to the UK from Canada via Maastricht in The Netherlands and there is a huge amount of educational research about it. If you are interested, try putting 'PBL' into a PubMed search.

Step (jump) 1: Clarifying terms

This is an interesting step. The group reads through the problem statement, which is often a paragraph or more, and identify any words or phrases that anyone in the group does not understand fully. Either other members of the group can help provide a definition or the group can list the word or statement as something that they will need to look up. Clearly, this is an important step because the group needs to have the same understanding of the words in the problem to be able to discuss it, but in addition, in some research at Bart's and the London and Kings, we have found that this stage seems to help allow students to feel safe to admit 'not knowing' right at the beginning of the session. This was valued and felt to be different from a tutor-led tutorial.

Step 2: Define the issues

In this step, the students try and list as many issues as they can see in the problem – perhaps 'What is diabetes? Why was this patient started on insulin? What would have happened if she hadn't had treatment? Why didn't she take her insulin as prescribed?' and so on. There are often main issues and sub-issues, sometimes there are a number of different angles (perhaps a biomedical, a sociological, a legal perspective).

Note that many texts use the word 'problems' rather than 'issues' for this step, but we have noticed that this can cause confusion between the initial problem ('problem statement') and then breaking that down into further 'problems', if you see what we mean. We will stick with 'issues' for clarity.

Step 3: Brainstorm/analyse the issues

Here the group takes each issue in turn and brainstorms freely on what they know about it. Personal experience, prior knowledge, even hunches are fine. The brainstorm does not need to be structured, it is just about making an inventory of the group's knowledge. You might remember from Chapter 2 that new knowledge is linked to old knowledge in the long-term memory and that for deep learning to occur that old knowledge, 'prior knowledge', needs to be activated. There is a fair amount of evidence that this step really does lead to better retention of facts later. The scribe aims to capture all these thoughts on the board and a good chairperson will make sure that they manage, by summarising, guiding and preventing everyone from talking at once.

Step 4: Organise ideas

Here the group, often with a lot of help from the scribe, look at the knowledge that they have on the board and try and make sense of it, often by clustering information together. The 'issues' tend to be ignored here, and the information is reorganised, to build hypotheses. This helps link and integrate

Chapter 5

knowledge across domains, which has been shown to improve retention and recall. Interestingly, even if the hypotheses are wrong, when students later (in step 6) discover that they are wrong, they still learn the right things much better than if they had just read the books without trying to get their thoughts together first. So, even if the group doesn't know much about the topic, it is still worthwhile persevering with steps 3 and 4.

Step 5: Generating learning objectives

Step 4 will reveal some areas that the group are strong in, that they are sure of, and will also reveal gaps. In our example, the group might well know what diabetes is and how it is defined and diagnosed, but they might realise that they are unable to explain how glucose causes all the complications of diabetes at the cellular/molecular level, they might be uncertain of what all the possible complications of diabetes are and they might realise that they are curious about how people adapt to a new diagnosis of diabetes and what factors help and hinder a positive adaptation. They have, therefore, generated four learning objectives. They might fine-tune these to be more specific so that everyone is sure what they will be required to answer when they next meet. Often the facilitator (tutor) will have a hidden agenda of some areas that need to be covered for the curriculum.

As a group or as an individual you might generate extra objectives, above and beyond what is expected; perhaps you are interested or curious about something or perhaps your discussions identified a gap in your knowledge that you need to fill.

Step 6: Self-study

Students study for all objectives on their own. They usually read more widely, but the objectives that they generated guide their study and at the least they should be able to answer all the objectives that they had agreed as a group. Sources might include books, journal articles and other formal learning materials. More subjective sources might have some value too – expert opinion (including clinicians, patients) and, of course, the Internet – but these sources should be used sparingly. As always, be careful with the Internet – see Chapter 2, p. 39 for some tips on judging the quality of a website. Ideally, you should look at a wide variety of sources and evaluate/triangulate what they say.

Step 7: Reporting back

This step usually happens a few days or a week later. It has the same chair and the same scribe. Often it starts with students going round saying where they found their information. Then each learning objective is taken in turn and the group explain it, often with one student taking a lead for each objectives.

If you have a good facilitator, they might ask you sideways questions (perhaps how you would apply your new knowledge to a slightly different situation) to help you elaborate your knowledge and to help you to identify whether you really have understood it as much as you thought you had.

Even though you will have done all your homework on your own, this step helps you learn through teaching/explaining, it also helps you learn through questioning and applying. It allows you to measure the depth and breadth of knowledge that you have learnt against your peers and is fantastic for motivation.

Making problem-based learning work for you

We have written quite a bit about PBL, and in doing so, we hope that you can witness two clear messages that are often misunderstood. First, the process is not about generating objectives, it is about maximising subsequent learning and recall. Some institutions actually give the suggested objectives at the beginning of the session and the students still benefit in terms of relevance, motivation and learning from going through the process. Unfortunately, this approach is rare and the hidden nature of the objectives often makes them seem the only important thing. (*'We had a great PBL session: we got the objectives out of it in 10 minutes flat'* could be translated as *'We cheated ourselves out of an opportunity for deep learning, and our tutor didn't stop us'*.)

Our second point is simple; everything that you read in the first half of this chapter applies here. PBL is simply a structured way of going about group work. If you think about the things we covered in the first half of this chapter, and how they influence the way the group works, you will be two-thirds of the way for producing a more productive group.

Study groups

Study groups tend to be groups that students set up themselves in order to learn. Some are more formal than others, but the productive ones tend to follow rules, whether spoken out loud or unwritten. There are usually ground rules about behaviour.

Clinical skills and clinical communication skills

We have discussed how students' own study groups can help development of skills in Chapters 3 and 4. Remember that to learn any skill you need to know how to do it, you need to practise and you need feedback. And all this within the spotlight of the learner's frame of mind (motivation, self belief etc). The three key messages that we want to highlight here are ensuring that your learning is active learning, giving and receiving feedback, and managing your own and your group's frame of mind. Active learning takes two forms: either doing (and you need to practise to learn; however much you watch someone else perform figure skating, you will not be able to do it unless you practise on the ice) or by actively observing. You can learn a lot from watching someone else perform a skill that you are learning – watch attentively and think about what you are learning from doing so. There is no point in being there if you cannot see what is going on. Feedback is, of course, essential. Giving constructive feedback (as opposed to destructive feedback, pointless feedback or no feedback) to the other members of your group will help them learn and will keep the group together. Be sure that you are willing to receive feedback from your peers too – ask for it and pursue it until you get the feedback that you need.

In chapter 3 (clinical skills), you thought about how your learning of clinical skills are affected by your motivation for the topic and for medicine in general, your beliefs about that particular topic ('it's just too difficult'), your beliefs about yourself ('I can never learn lists') and your response to failure ('I am too stupid'). Of course, all the same goes for group learning. One of your tasks is to monitor and, if necessary, challenge negative outlooks.

Interprofessional education

As a doctor, you will be expected to work closely with other professions – nurses, physiotherapists, dieticians, midwives – the list is a long one. Many medical schools introduce some interprofessional learning, often in small groups, within their curricula to try and help students prepare for interprofessional working later on in life. The aim of such sessions is to help you learn 'with, from and about each other', and on paper they seem like a great idea. In practice, it can be touch and go whether such sessions are useful or not.

In her review of interprofessional education (IPE), Della Freeth (2007) argues convincingly that IPE is simply 'a special case of professional education so knowledge about good practice in learning and teaching in a wide range of contexts can be applied directly to IPE', and we agree. To make IPE work, you can apply the contents of this chapter, just as with any other form of group work. If you are aware of roles within the group, of how the group dynamic develops and how you can help it grow, if you pay attention to the behaviours within the group, and are truly curious about other people's point of view and all the other things that we have covered, then IPE will work well for you.

Summary

Studying, learning and working in a group is essential, and there are many different advantages to doing so. Indeed, some medical school's entire curriculum is based on group work. There are also challenges along the way. In this chapter, we have tried to highlight the following factors, which are under your influence, to help you make group work for you. They apply across any and every form of group work. You will not get it right every time, but we believe strongly that if you are aware of these factors, you reflect on them and invest some perseverance that you will succeed.

- Roles within the group: do you have a good spread? If not, what can you do about it?
- Development of group dynamic: how can you ease the group through the stages to start performing?
- Goals: Are your goals concrete enough? Are they shared? Do they help encourage or discourage collaboration?
- Individual factors: Are you all at a reasonably similar level? Do you appreciate each other's knowledge and skills?
- Behaviours: Does the group ask questions, build links, elaborate knowledge? How about cognitive conflict and debate – is it welcomed? How structured is the process – would more structure help? Are different points of view valued? What does the group do to maximise motivation in its members?

References and further reading

We based much of the educational psychology of collaborative learning on the following papers and texts.

Belbin, R. M. (1981). *Management Teams: Why They Succeed or Fail*. London, Heinemann.

Boxtel, C., van der Linden, J., Kanselaar, G. *et al.* (2000). *Deep Processing in a Collaborative Learning Environment. Social Interaction in Learning and Instruction: the meaning of discourse for the construction of knowledge*. Amsterdam, Pergamom.

Freeth, D. (2007). *Interprofessional Education*. Edinburgh, Association for the Student of Medical Education.

Novak, J. D. (2002). Meaningful learning: the essential factor for conceptual change in limited or inappropriate prepositional hierarchies leading to empowerment of learners. *Science Education, 86*, 548–571.

Slavin, R. E. (1996). Research on cooperative learning and achievement: what we know, what we need to know. *Contemporary Educational Psychology, 21*, 43–69.

Watkins, B. & Gibson-Sweet, M. (1997). Sailing with Belbin. *Education and Training 39*, 105–110.

Westberg, J. & Jason, H. (1996). *Fostering Learning in Small Groups: A Practical Guide*. New York, Springer Publishing Company.

If you find you have quite a lot of difficulty working in a group, Stella Cottrell's book gives quite a nice practical guide on simple behaviours that can help build confidence and skills:

Cottrell, S. (2003). *The Study Skills Handbook*. Basingstoke, Palgrave Macmillan.

An entry level article on problem-based learning, well worth digging out of the dusty basement of your library is:

Schmidt, H. G. (1993). Foundations of problem-based learning: some explanatory notes. *Medical Education, 27*, 422–432.

Questions and answers

Q: I cannot work in a group – to be brutally honest, there is no one I really like in my year, no one that I really want to spend time with. I am a mature student and all my friends are from outside medical school.

A: This is a common area of confusion. You do not need to marry people that you study with. They do not need to be your friends. Indeed, sometimes it helps if they are not – especially if you tend to lark about with your friends.

Q: Everyone in my group keeps shouting each other down, we seem to get nowhere, what can I do?

A: This might be a normal stage of development of a group, so if it is a one-off, perhaps you should just hang in there. If it has been going on for a while, have you discussed this in the group? Perhaps you could agree some simple ground rules (see previously). You might want to seek out some expert advice from a respected, experienced facilitator in the medical school; they are bound to have some tips that will help.

Q: I hate IPE, what is the point? What could I learn from a nurse?

A: We know that most major medical errors occur when different health professionals do not communicate effectively and work together; therefore, if you think that there is no point communicating effectively with different professions, then medicine is probably not for you. It is not easy though, it requires a commitment to try and understand someone else's point of view and a large amount of on-going effort. The desired outcome is excellent patient care through good interprofessional team working, and with this end in sight, the point becomes clearer.

Q: Not much group work happens in my medical school, how can I convince people to get a group together?

A: Lots of people in your year will be feeling the same as you right now. You might want to summarise the start of this chapter (the pros and cons) and talk to those around you. The fact that the whole is greater than the sum of its parts might be a particularly good selling point. Having and communicating a clear structure for the first sessions and a clearly understood objective that people can prepare for will make those first few sessions more likely to succeed – then the ball will be rolling!

Chapter 6 **Developing your academic writing skills**

OVERVIEW

This chapter provides a brief introduction to academic writing. We describe the importance of planning when writing and highlight some potential pitfalls, particularly with respect to referencing and plagiarism.

Introduction

Writing well is a key skill for a doctor; developing this skill now will stand you in good stead for writing educational materials, research articles, patient information leaflets and even the odd book chapter. Your school will run academic writing courses; you should make an effort to go to one of these courses and apply what you learn as quickly as possible. This section gives a brief introduction to writing an essay, but is not intended to replace some expert tutoring. You will find whole books on how to write an essay in your library; we reference some in the further reading section of this chapter, and it would be worthwhile reading one.

Most of the academic writing that you are asked to do at medical school will be set assignments that you write in your own time – either as essays or as reflective commentaries (for your portfolio, for example) or other documents. In this chapter, we will specifically refer to essays, but the same principles apply to the other forms of academic writing. There are some simple steps to go through to help you construct a winning essay, and in the next couple of pages, we have tried to identify one approach.

How to Succeed at Medical School: An Essential Guide to Learning, Second Edition.
Dason Evans and Jo Brown.
© 2015 John Wiley & Sons, Ltd. Published 2015 by John Wiley & Sons, Ltd.

I really found it difficult to get my thoughts and ideas down on paper in a way that others appreciated. The course that my library ran really helped me to do this.

Jumaane, first-year medical student.

Collecting information

If you have read the section on note taking (Chapter 2), you will see lots of techniques that you can use here. You will first either collect your existing notes together and decide what is relevant to the essay or search sources afresh for the essay. Try and do all the searching and reading you need *before* you start the essay, as otherwise you might not realise that the whole focus needs to change until you are halfway through writing. Crucially, remember to record your sources so that you can reference them appropriately. Use your own words to make notes, and if you write down any direct quotes, put them in quotation marks in your notes so that you know that you will need to treat them as direct quotes in your essay.

Organise all your information in one place, perhaps as a concept map or MindMap and look for themes that answer the question. Look also for contrasting information that you might highlight as an area of uncertainty.

The message(s)

Decide on what the key points are that you want to cover and decide in what order you would like them to occur. Often there will be one or two key, central messages that you want to get across. In this book, for example, the key messages that we are trying to get across are that the student is the most important person in the learning process; that learning how to learn is an active process which requires deliberate practice and that knowing how you learn (metacognition) results in better outcomes.

Your message may be very clear to you – perhaps you want to argue that drug company advertising should be banned or perhaps that improving communication skills in doctors will save money on patient care – try and choose an interesting key message, something with a slant. You can then use your essay to explain both sides of the argument and through this to justify your stance.

Constructing an overview

You might construct your overview using a flow chart, some sentences or even adapt your concept map from your notes. The patchwork method can also be used, where you make a box for each section of the essay and write key points within each box. You might start the whole process off with a brainstorming session: annotate the session from your reading, organise it in order to answer the question and then further annotate it to make a detailed paragraph plan.

However you go about it, most essays will be divided up into an introduction, a body, conclusions and references. The body might be further subdivided either explicitly using headings (this approach being more common in the sciences) or implicitly using the paragraph contents (more common in the arts).

Make sure that you keep looking back at the question or topic throughout the writing of your essay and especially at the overview stage (Figure 6.1). It is easy to get sidetracked into answering a different question to the one that you were given.

> *The trick to writing an essay is to spend plenty of time planning it; working out what goes where, that makes the writing easy.*
>
> Roger, fourth-year medical student.

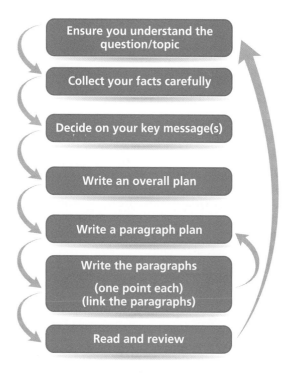

Figure 6.1   Overview of essay writing.

The paragraphs

You should now have planned the different sections, the things that you want to cover in each section and the order that you wish to cover them. It is time to start writing. In general, one idea should go in one paragraph. Often this will form the first sentence of the paragraph and the rest of the text will elaborate on it (although in this paragraph the key point has arrived only in the third sentence). This rule of thumb will make it easier for the reader to see your main arguments and their justification.

Unfortunately, this approach can come across as a little disjointed, so think about adding a 'link' sentence at the end of one paragraph or at the start of the next. You might, for example, see the first half of the first sentence of this paragraph as a link between these two paragraphs. If your two paragraphs cannot link together, then you probably need to go back to your plan and see if you need to rearrange the order that the key points come in, in order to produce a more fluent document.

> *My tutor told me that my paragraphs were all over the place, she showed me how I could change their order to make a story flow better, and add a sentence here and there to link them together. I was really impressed at the finished product!*
>
> Ingrid, intercalated BSc student.

Examples of link sentences at the end of a paragraph or start of the next might include the following:

- 'However, this opinion is not shared by all authors.' Next paragraph: 'Roger Lewis (1993) argues that . . .'
- 'Of course, syphilis is not the only cause of wart-like growths around the anus.' Next paragraph 'Genital warts were first described in . . .'
- '. . . in this way, Wilson felt he had proven the cause of diabetes.' Next paragraph: 'Many other authors at this time also considered that diabetes was caused by an imbalance of the humours . . .'
- Next paragraph: 'These changes have resulted in . . .'

Back to the drawing board

Depending how much of an obsessive planner you are, you might find that new themes or realisations occur to you while you are writing. If this happens, you should go back to your plan and see how it fits in; you might need to move your paragraphs around to build a new argument for your new point.

Start at the middle, end with the start

In general, it is useful to end by writing the introduction, which provides the necessary background, relevance and lays out the main arguments, and then finally with the conclusions, which should draw the whole essay together.

Active or passive

One of the dilemmas in academic writing is whether to write it in an active or passive style. Passive styles seem more 'academic' and yet there is considerable evidence that active styles are more readable. Consider the following two introductions:

Communication skills are essential to professional life as a doctor. In this essay I will demonstrate from the literature that poor communication skills result in significant costs, not only in terms of worse patient outcomes and in terms of litigation, but also in terms of a social cost to the population as a whole and the trust that it puts in doctors. I will then describe the wide body of evidence that shows that clinical communication skills can be improved through training and will go on to argue for the benefits of mandatory training of doctors in clinical communication skills including its cost-effectiveness.

or

Communication skills are essential to professional life as a doctor. In this paper the evidence from the literature will be explored to demonstrate that poor communication skills result in significant costs, not only in terms of worse patient outcomes and in terms of litigation but also in terms of a social cost to the population as a whole and the trust that it puts in doctors. A wide body of evidence will be reviewed, showing that clinical communication skills can be improved through training and finally a clear argument will be built that the benefits of mandatory training of doctors in clinical communication skills are considerable and would represent a cost-effective intervention.

The first introduction represented an active style ('I will demonstrate'), the second introduction a passive style ('the evidence . . . will be explored'). Experiment with both approaches and ask your tutors if there is a preferred style in your school. Hopefully, the first introduction demonstrates to you that an active style can be used and still make a compelling academic argument.

Plagiarism and referencing

Plagiarism

Plagiarism and referencing is not a focus of the book, but deserves a mention here. If you write down someone else's ideas, you *must* acknowledge them through referencing, otherwise you are passing them off as your ideas and that is academically dishonest (and is seen by many as equivalent to stealing and lying at the same time). This is why writing down your sources when making notes is so important – so that you know where the ideas came from. If you directly copy someone's words, it must be *completely* clear that these are their words and not yours; usually you will use quotation marks for this, in addition to referencing. In general, it is seen as inappropriate to copy large chunks of text from another source even if you do use quotation marks and references.

Referencing is not only used to demonstrate that you are honest and to acknowledge the 'owner' of the ideas that you use, you should also use references to justify key and controversial points in your essays and to demonstrate that you have synthesised the literature to inform your points rather than just written down your random opinions.

Note that we suggest that when you are writing an essay, you collect all the information you plan to use in one place first, by making notes in your own words and including some explicit linkage in your notes to the source of information (some people write one large index card for each reference, with the name and detail of the source at the top of the card, others use concept maps with the reference as the root or centre or stem of the map). We then suggest that you try to pick out a message and justify it from these authors. This method makes it easy to avoid plagiarism.

In contrast, imagine the student who writes his or her essay directly from several sources, the books or web pages open in front of him. The temptation will be not to think, not to synthesise and critique the literature and not to build an argument, but rather just to copy out one paragraph from here and one paragraph from there. Not only does the resulting essay look terrible, but the student is suddenly in major trouble for plagiarism.

There are two main forms of referencing: the first is an author–date format when the name and date is inserted in the text as the reference. The proper name for this type of referencing is the Harvard style and, to confuse things, there are various different subtypes. Basically, you put the name of the author and the year that they published the paper you are referencing in the body of the text and the full details of their paper, book or website reference at the end in alphabetical order. Examples of usage include the following:

In their paper on preparedness for practice, Evans and colleagues (2004) highlighted feelings of high anxiety in newly qualified doctors.

Anxiety is common in newly qualified doctors (Evans, 2004) …

In contrast to Harvard style (author–date), the Vancouver approach uses numbers to link to references at the end of the text. Depending on which flavour of Vancouver is being used, the number may be a superscript,[1] or in the text in a round bracket (2) or a square bracket [3]. The *British Medical Journal* uses the superscript approach. Examples include the following:

In their paper on preparedness for practice, Evans and colleagues[1] highlighted feelings of high anxiety in newly qualified doctors.

Anxiety is common in newly qualified doctors.[1]

Unfortunately, every different form or flavour of referencing has a slightly different format, especially of the references at the end of your paper. Unless you invest in some software that helps referencing or your school provides this for free (check with your library, you might be surprised), it is probably best to stick to 'pure Harvard' format for all your essays (the name and date help you remember what you read where) or 'pure Vancouver' if your school requires you to use a numbered style. A discussion with your library or even a simple web search (try the following in a search engine – 'citation style Harvard') will provide you with all the information that you need to reference appropriately.

Learning more

This book does not demonstrate referencing well; it would not rate highly as an academic piece of literature. Most of the text is written from experience and years of working with students, many of them struggling. When we specifically use ideas from other authors we reference explicitly and when we have turned to several similar texts to make sure that what we are writing is reasonable we cite them as references and further reading. Journal articles are the opposite extreme, ensuring often that every point that they make can be referenced to the wider literature. Have a look at some articles in one of the major journals as examples of referencing, you never know, you might get a taste for reading the journals on a regular basis.

In addition to pointing you towards useful resources, your medical library will run fantastic courses on plagiarism and referencing; go to one early in your course and consider going again a year or two later. These are fundamental academic skills that will last you a lifetime.

Summary

Although academic writing is becoming a less common activity on medical courses, being able to communicate clearly in a written form is an essential skill for a doctor. Assignments that require academic writing give you a fantastic opportunity to demonstrate your understanding of the complexities around a topic. More is required than just writing, and good preparation by way of searching for information and planning the key messages and

Chapter 6

detailed structure of the essay before you start writing will result in much more chance of success.

References and further reading

Your library is likely to have a wide variety of books on essay writing and a huge training resource around referencing and plagiarism. As we have already mentioned, a web search is also likely to be fruitful. You might find some of the following references useful.

Cottrell, S. (2006). *The Exam Skills Handbook: Achieving Peak Performance*. Basingstoke, Palgrave Macmillan.

Evans, M. (2004). *How to Pass Exams Every Time*. Oxford, How To Books.

Lewis, R. S. (1993). *How to Write Essays*. London, National Extension College.

Pears, R. & Shields, G. (2005). *Cite them Right: The Essential Guide to Referencing and Plagiarism*. Newcastle, Pear Tree Books.

Questions and answers

Q: If I paraphrase something from the book, then it is not plagiarism, right?

A: Wrong. If you use someone else's ideas, you must reference them, whether they are their words or not.

Q: I think I have dyslexia; as I find writing essays so difficult, what should I do?

A: Dyslexia is only one of a range of specific learning difficulties, so expert advice would be advised. You should talk this through with your personal tutor and they may well be able to organise for you to have an assessment at your university's learning unit. While this is underway, or even if you do have a diagnosis, you may want to concentrate even harder on planning essays and assignments in the way that we have explained. You might find more visual representations, such a MindMap and flow charts, useful in your planning.

Q: My tutor has asked me to write up my project for publication – Help!

A: In addition to the advice in this chapter, have a look at some articles in the journal that you are aiming for to get a feel for the style and structure required. Make a first stab at it (spending particular attention to planning and to referencing) and meet with your tutor. If they have published before then their mentoring will be a great learning experience for you. Do not forget to put them as a co-author on the first draft.

Chapter 7 **Portfolios and reflection**

OVERVIEW

Portfolios are increasingly popular in both undergraduate and postgraduate medical education. Chances are that as a medical student, junior doctor and specialist, you will be required to keep a portfolio up to date and you will be assessed on that portfolio. As you will see in this chapter, portfolios are more than just collections of information, and they include reflections and often formal reflective commentaries. Students sometimes struggle with the concept of reflection, so we have added a brief section introducing a model for practical reflection.

Introduction

Different institutions use portfolios for different purposes and in different formats, so, not surprisingly, there is often quite a bit of confusion as to what a portfolio is and more than a little resentment and negative feelings about them. This chapter aims to clear up some of the mysteries around portfolios and to help you see how to make a portfolio work in your favour. Because of the wide variety in formats of portfolios, we will try and keep most of the advice as generic as possible, with some specific examples to show you how you might apply this advice to your situation. As with the other chapters in this book, you will need to actively engage with the content in order to benefit.

What is a portfolio?

A portfolio is a personal collection of information relating to your professional development. More than just containing a record of facts, it is a dynamic and changing document that records and directs your reflections and progress as a medical student and beyond.

How to Succeed at Medical School: An Essential Guide to Learning, Second Edition.
Dason Evans and Jo Brown.
© 2015 John Wiley & Sons, Ltd. Published 2015 by John Wiley & Sons, Ltd.

What is a portfolio useful for?

From your personal perspective, portfolios are useful for collecting, reflecting and planning. From the perspective of those above you, portfolios are also used for assessing and making judgements.

Imagine that at the start of medical school, you buy a big folder and as a front sheet you list the General Medical Council's (GMC) duties of a doctor (Box 7.1). You buy one of those 12-piece dividers so that you have a section for each of the GMC's six main categories. In each of the four sections, you keep information that you gather under that heading. Under 'Provide a good standard of practice and care', for example, you might keep a record of your exam results and under 'Protect and promote the health of patients and the public', you might keep a record of some health promotion teaching that you went to in the first year and the community health project that you completed in the third year. Imagine that at finals, the GMC asks you to demonstrate that you have reached the criteria required for graduation, and you get out your folder (or by then several folders) and show them that you can demonstrate that you fulfil all the duties of a doctor already, your discussions with the GMC would be very easy.

Portfolios tend to be more than a collection of evidence. They tend to include reflections too. Perhaps you will use some of the spare sections in your folder to add a commentary or ongoing reflection on the evidence that you submit. What, for example, did you learn from the health promotion teaching that you went to in the first year? In what way will it change your practice? How will you know? What did your last set of exam results tell you? What do you need to do as a result? How will you know that you have made the improvements that you decided on?

You might decide to include not only glowing examples under each of the sections but also some things that do not go so well. Perhaps in your first year, you are disciplined for plagiarism (Chapter 6) and nearly lose your place in medical school. You might include this under the 'honesty' section and write a reflective commentary on what you learned from the whole experience. Writing a reflective log will help you think about this in a structured way.

By way of helping you plan, imagine that you look through your folder on a regular basis and you decide that under 'Keep your professional knowledge and skills up to date' you cross-reference with the list of skills in one of the GMC's other documents, *Tomorrow's Doctors* (GMC, 2009), and you realise that although they list competence in passing a urethral catheter as a core skill requirement for a new doctor, you have not done many/any. You therefore find an opportunity to practise in the skills laboratory and then arrange (with every ounce of charm that you have) to go out on the wards with the urology nurse practitioner, watch him or her in action and then give it a go

Box 7.1 The duties of a doctor registered with the General Medical Council (from Good Medical Practice (2013))
The duties of a doctor registered with the General Medical Council
Patients must be able to trust doctors with their lives and health. To justify that trust you must show respect for human life and make sure your practice meets the standards expected of you in four domains.

Knowledge, skills and performance
- Make the care of your patient your first concern.
- Provide a good standard of practice and care.
  - Keep your professional knowledge and skills up to date.
  - Recognise and work within the limits of your competence.

Safety and quality
- Take prompt action if you think that patient safety, dignity or comfort is being compromised.
- Protect and promote the health of patients and the public.

Communication, partnership and teamwork
- Treat patients as individuals and respect their dignity.
  - Treat patients politely and considerately.
  - Respect patients' right to confidentiality.
- Work in partnership with patients.
  - Listen to, and respond to, their concerns and preferences.
  - Give patients the information they want or need in a way they can understand.
  - Respect patients' right to reach decisions with you about their treatment and care.
  - Support patients in caring for themselves to improve and maintain their health.
- Work with colleagues in the ways that best serve patients' interests.

Maintaining trust
- Be honest and open and act with integrity.
- Never discriminate unfairly against patients or colleagues.
- Never abuse your patients' trust in you or the public's trust in the profession.
You are personally accountable for your professional practice and must always be prepared to justify your decisions and actions.

on a suitably consenting patient. You keep practising until you are competent and confident. Your portfolio has helped identify a weakness and has helped you plan to address it.

A lot of the learning that you will do in medical school will be through reflections on your interactions with patients in clinical settings. Did things go as expected, or not? Why? What were the strengths and weaknesses of your communication with the patient? Did you miss a key sign on clinical examination? Perhaps you felt that you had failed to build rapport with the patient. A reflective commentary in your portfolio allows you to deconstruct what happened and plan what you might do differently next time, even stimulate you to look some things up.

A portfolio is, therefore, clearly useful to you in terms of collecting evidence, reflecting on and learning from it, and in terms of helping you plan how to fill any gaps in your knowledge or skills. The use of portfolios as an assessment tool is, however, more controversial. Portfolios can clearly be assessed on the quantity and range of evidence that you have collected, but also they can be assessed in terms of the reflections that you have made – do you look like someone who really thinks about what happens (good or bad) and really tries to learn from it?

The real secret of portfolios is to make the portfolio your own. Initially ignore what everyone else tells you and spend some time thinking about what you want a portfolio for – what will be the focus for you. How would it look? What would be the headings? How often would you look at it? Only after you have an idea of the answers, you should go back and look at what the school is asking you to do. Work towards a compromise – something that you own and want – that will also do what the school wants for you too.

The basic structure of a portfolio

There are a thousand different variations on 'portfolio', but depending who you speak to either all or most have a similar structure (Figure 7.1): all have a list of headings or topics which might be called **goals** or outcomes. These might be as specific as a list of clinical skills that you need to master or as open-ended as the GMC duties of a doctor in the aforementioned example. They might be as impersonal as something your school has set for you or as personal as something from your heart. Perhaps one of your goals might relate to enjoying your social life more.

This list of goals or outcomes is linked to **evidence** that you collect, which will reside in folders sections or under headings. You will probably start with a little evidence from secondary school, perhaps some certificates and exam results, and will build up from there. Of course, one piece of evidence may relate to several goals, so there is usually some indexing or cross-referencing. For example, you may have two goals, one relating to developing a broad anatomy knowledge and the other relating to pursuing a career as a surgeon. Your high mark in a surgical anatomy exam might cross-reference to both goals.

```
┌─────────────────────────────────────────────────┐
│                                                 │
│  Goals                                          │
│                                                 │
│  Evidence                                       │
│                                                 │
│  Reflective commentary (What did you learn?     │
│  Where are the gaps?)                           │
│                                                 │
│  Action plan                                    │
│                                                 │
└─────────────────────────────────────────────────┘
```

Figure 7.1 Structure of a portfolio.

In addition to the evidence, you will need to write some sort of **reflective commentary** on the evidence; this might include reflection on the evidence itself (what did you learn from doing the community health project?), on how this evidence moves you closer to fulfilling your goals (and what gaps are left that still need to be filled?) or both. These reflections may generate an **action plan** for change. The concept of 'reflection' is often a puzzle to medical students. Later in this chapter, we cover it in more depth.

Special cases: e-portfolios

Paper-based portfolios are reasonably easy to imagine – a folder with sections containing goals, evidence and reflections. e-Portfolios can be trickier to visualise, but still contain the same structure. An electronic or web-based portfolio has some advantages. It is easy for storage (you do not need to carry around huge folders), and if you choose a web-based version, it can be accessible from anywhere in the world. You can even have different levels of access; you might allow your tutor to see some parts, but perhaps not some of your more personal reflections. For these reasons, in addition to the trend factor, the use of e-portfolios is rapidly expanding in medical schools and beyond it into postgraduate education.

> IT is my thing, and as I'm webmaster for a student society I thought I had to have an online portfolio, and I found a really good one that was free too. One of my tutors needed some help navigating it, but when I had sat with him and showed him how it works, he thought it was fantastic!
>
> Faruq, fourth-year medical student.

You should note some cautions before leaping wholeheartedly into a paper-free portfolio.

- Importantly you should consider the longevity of the portfolio – if your medical school are offering you an e-portfolio, what will happen when you graduate? Will you be able to keep the data and access to it? Imagine that you suddenly have 5 or 6 years' worth of information, all cross-referenced in a nice multidimensional way, not designed to print out, and you have to leave it all behind and try and translate it to some kind of written one or some other electronic version when you leave medical school.
- You might also think about how others will access your portfolio and if there might be some online access or a useful way of printing out relevant parts. Will it be private and secure enough to keep pranksters away and yet allow access to those you want?
- The structure of the portfolio is much more open for innovation if all the information is electronic, but be aware that it can rapidly become quite complex and difficult to navigate. You will need to spend time on a regular basis reviewing the structure and adjusting it as necessary.
- Remember that you will still get a lot of evidence in hard copy form – certificates and so forth. You can, perhaps, scan these in if you have access to a scanner, but remember that if it is a high stakes portfolio, you will need to keep the original documents somewhere safe too.

This is not to say anything against online portfolios, but rather to encourage you to think about what you want out of the portfolio and how you should structure it before you spend considerable time, effort and perhaps money on something that turns out not to be as useful as you had imagined.

Perhaps the most exciting aspect of e-portfolios is where they will go next: integration into wikis, blogs (why not keep your reflections as a blog anyway?), social networking sites, directly linking to journals and search engines and so on. The next few years will be exciting, and you might be a pioneer: be prepared to experiment and share what works, and especially what does not! Before putting reflections online, have a look at chapter 13 on professionalism, and particularly digital professionalism.

Making your portfolio work for you

There are only two rules for making a portfolio useful: you should feel complete ownership of your portfolio, and you should review it regularly. The portfolio should be yours, and yours alone, and you should design it and build it and maintain it for your own benefit. Perhaps you will start one now, using goals that you have generated from this book. One goal might be to develop more effective study skills. You might write a reflective commentary considering how broad and deep your toolkit of study skills currently is, and where you want to develop over the next year. Following on from that you might generate a plan for the next year – to practise using keywords and concept maps for your learning for 3 months, to attend a study skills workshop at your university and to start a study group with some colleagues from medical school. In a couple of months, you can see how far you are down that line, if you have collected any evidence and if it demonstrates progress. You are using this portfolio to drive your own progress.

> *My portfolio is mine, I love it, I spent time making it beautiful and I really enjoy just looking through it, it shows me a map of where I have been and where I am going.*
>
> Mina, third-year medical student.

It seems that most humans (not just students) tend to run rather close to deadlines. Non-urgent things are put to the bottom of the pile whereas more urgent things always get put on top. The temptation will be to neglect your portfolio, and you may need to make particular effort not to. Perhaps you could timetable some time every week or fortnight just to file evidence, flick through it, consider where you are (from the evidence) in moving towards your goals (goals), what you have learnt from the evidence and how you are progressing (reflections); you might even write down a paragraph of your thoughts and sometimes you might realise that you need to change direction (action plan). Regular review will mean that your portfolio is always current, always relevant and that it is *alive*. Doing a little, often, will ensure that if anyone wants to see your portfolio or if you need to dip into it to produce some evidence, no additional effort will be required.

Many of your peers will see portfolios as a nuisance, they will not contribute regularly to them and they will frantically try and complete 12 months' worth of information the night before a portfolio review. Their reflections will be largely fictitious and they will moan about what a 'pointless chore' portfolios are. They are right, *their* portfolio will be pointless but make sure that yours is not.

Assessment of portfolios

We have already mentioned that there are different approaches to assessing (marking) portfolios. Some institutions just require that a portfolio is kept, others mark on the collection of evidence – perhaps the quantity (consultants are often assessed on the total number of hours of staff development activity that they have completed) or the breadth (are you fulfilling a wide range of goals to become a rounded doctor?). These assessments are relatively easy to design and mark. Some medical schools also mark on the quality of the reflective commentaries. The hope is that this will drive students to reflect often and result in graduates who can really deconstruct experiences and learn from them. Unfortunately, it also drives some students to produce outstanding works of reflective fiction.

If your school marks on the quality of the reflective commentary, it is important to know that they are doing this to encourage you to reflect often. They will be looking for honest accounts, not only of how great you are, but also of where things have gone wrong, what you have learnt from these and how you are planning to improve. If you see the portfolio as belonging to you, and for your benefit, then what is the point of writing fiction, of cheating yourself?

Reflection

What is reflection?

Much has been written about reflection and there are many good books available that examine it in depth. The purpose of this section is to give you an overview and some simple tools to get you started with it quickly.

> *Our minds have two positions: looking out and looking in.*
>
> (Rinpoche, 1992)

Reflection is the **looking in**, a deep thinking technique that allows us to plan for or analyse events that have already happened and to extract maximum learning from them – a sort of 're-evaluation of experience' (Boud, 2006). Reflection helps to develop an extra level of consciousness or a 'third eye', which allows us to become more aware of our own part or the 'self' in any given situation. Reflective skills are an important part of personal and professional development for all health-care professionals and some authors argue that it is the main way we effectively learn from experience as adults. Reflecting honestly upon how you learn something or how a particular event has gone is a way of deconstructing experiences and learning from them – a way of learning for real understanding.

> *Reflection was boring, boring, boring until I realised it was just another way of thinking about what I do and making thinking work for me.*
>
> Gavin, third-year student.

We have already thought about the importance of finding out about your preferred personal learning styles in order to become an effective learner (Chapter 1). Developing reflective skills will also help you to develop your 'third eye' and give you the means to learn from all life events, so that everything is useful and valuable experiences are never wasted.

Some people are natural reflectors, they think about events that have happened, both good and bad and try to work out what went well, what did not and what their own part in each may have been. For a lot of us, however, these skills do not come naturally; we have to work at them and actively implement them into our everyday life. Like learning any new skills, it takes a few weeks or months to become comfortable with them, but eventually they become part of what we are and second nature.

The reflective cycle
To get started or consolidate your reflective skills, it may be helpful to have a practical model as shown in Figure 7.2.

This can be used as a way of guiding reflection about any event, but as an example of how reflection can be used to think about how you learn, we have mapped a learning experience on to the cycle.

Description: what happened?
'I went to a 1-hour lecture on the functions of the cranial nerves along with my whole year. I came away at the end of it having learned almost nothing

Chapter 7

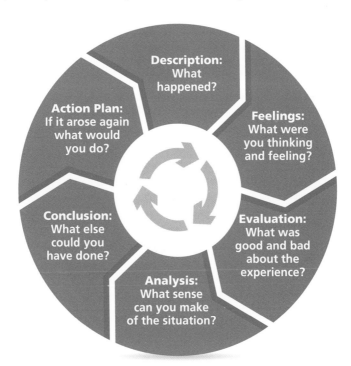

Figure 7.2   The reflective cycle (Gibbs, 1988).

and with confused and inadequate notes. There were not enough handouts for everyone and so I didn't even have these to fall back on. The whole lecture seemed like a waste of time for me.'

Feelings: what were you thinking and feeling?
'Even before the lecture some of my friends told me that cranial nerves are difficult to learn and yet always come up in exams. The lecturer also began the lecture by saying that this was a difficult subject and that people often fail it in exams. I felt nervous and apprehensive from the beginning and my confidence was low. I don't like lectures at the best of times and often find my mind wanders off and that I don't take good notes. I went home at the end feeling fed up and useless.'

Evaluation: what was good and bad about the experience?
'Lots of bad things, like I still don't know about cranial nerves and probably would fail any exam about them and that I find lectures so difficult. The good thing is that most of the others also find cranial nerves difficult, so I am not alone.'

Analysis: what sense can you make of the situation?
'I know that cranial nerves are important to know about and that I do need to understand them. I need to find a way of learning about them that is right for me. I think that my friends and the lecturer saying that they were difficult had a big influence on my learning and confidence in the lecture. I am more worried about failing exams than learning about cranial nerves!'

Conclusion: what else could you have done?
'I could have prepared for the lecture in advance so that the concepts were not new to me and perhaps made a diagram that could have been fleshed out during the lecture as a way of organising my notes. I think this would have made me more confident. I am going to sit nearer the front next time as it is too easy to let my mind wander when I sit at the back with the other dreamers! I could try recording the lecture to listen to later at home with my notes?'

Action plan: if it arose again what would you do?
'It will arise again as lectures happen frequently. I am determined to be in control in the future and not be influenced by what others say – friends and lecturers have their own motivations and agendas. I also want to discuss lectures in a group to make sure I understand everything and hear what other people have to say. My action plan:

- prepare for lectures to get a head start;
- prepare a rough diagram to shape my notes;
- be aware of my own feelings and how these can impede my learning;
- sit near the front;
- record the lecture;
- consolidate my learning in a group.

Many people reflect only on the negative or poor experiences, but it is important to reflect on the positive as well. Try applying the reflective cycle to a successful learning experience: establishing what went well and your part in it will be as valuable as what went wrong.

The reflective cycle can be applied to any situation – professional or private – to help analyse what happened, why and what you felt about it. Try applying it to a situation with friends or family or a patient encounter – it is very adaptable.

> *I find it hard to think about and reflect on difficult times when things have gone wrong because it's like going through the pain again. I do know though that I learn a lot from doing it.*
>
> Femi, fourth-year student.

Reflection as a preparation

Reflection can be used as a preparation for learning or for any event (Sully and Dallas, 2005). Consider the following scenario.

You are about to go on a new GP placement tomorrow. You probably have some ideas about what it will be like, particularly as you are a patient registered at a GP practice yourself! It is useful to think about these ideas and thoughts in preparation for the visit. Reflect upon these questions:

- What kind of patients do you think you will be meeting?
- What might be the main challenges to communicate with them?
- What common health problems might they present with?
- Will you be sitting in with the GP or talking to patients on your own?
- Will you be examining any patients?
- How do you feel about the placement?
- Which other health-care professionals will you be working with?
- How will you record your learning?

Your experience of being a patient will influence how you feel about the GP placement and it will be important to reflect on this. This process may help you to think of strategies for making the placement run smoothly so that it is a rich learning opportunity. After the placement, apply the reflective cycle model to analyse how things went and consolidate your learning.

Solo or group reflection?

People find different types of reflection helpful. Once it becomes part of your normal routine, you may find you naturally reflect at certain times of the day, for example, on the bus or in the shower. To begin with though, you may need to set aside regular times each day to get into the habit. Professor Parveen Kumar (author of one of the leading text books of medicine, past president of the BMA and world-renowned teacher) spends 15 minutes each night writing down a reflective log on what she has learned that day; what better role-model could you follow?

Solo

Some people find writing the best way to reflect and a good way of record-ing their thoughts so that they are not lost. Throughout history, people have kept diaries and these are really just informal reflective journals. A reflective journal can be helpful in returning to a subject to see if things have changed or as a reminder of events or experiences. Written reflection is also a valuable part of any personal and professional development portfolio and can be used to illustrate points or issues you are writing about. Sometimes re-reading a reflective journal can show how much progress you have made or how similar some experiences have been or that a pattern is emerging. Re-reading these after a period of years has elapsed is really interesting, and some authors have even used these as a basis for an autobiography!

Group

Reflecting in a group can be a fascinating way of deconstructing an event or learning experience and will not only provide valuable insight, but also the different perspectives and feelings of everyone else in the group. These can sometimes be so different from your own that it is a real eye-opener and a way of capturing a much wider view. This sort of group reflective process is sometimes developed further into a critical incident review, when a particular event needs to be analysed and investigated by a whole team as a means of problem solving and is often used by the NHS and other industries.

Summary

Portfolios and reflections go hand in hand. Portfolios provide a place for you to plan your goals, collect evidence to see that you are reaching your goals, learn from your experiences by reflection and actively plan. Reflection is a structured tool that allows you to learn from experience and can be used not only in portfolios, but anywhere. We have looked at the definition and applications of reflection in this section and applied these to a learning situation.

- Portfolios are used widely in medical education and come in many different forms.
- Generally, they contain goals, evidence, reflective commentaries and action plans.
- Portfolios can really help you be in charge of your own development, which is hugely motivating. Make sure that your portfolio is your own, and review and add to it regularly to make best use of it.
- Reflection is a way of learning about the world.
- Reflection can be used as a tool for thinking about and learning from *any* situation.
- Reflection can be used to prepare for situations.

References and further reading

Boud, D. (2006). The role of work-related learning in developing clinical and communication skills. *CETL Maximising Learning in Practice Conference.* (12 December, 2006) Bart's and the London, Queen Mary's School of Medicine and Dentistry.
General Medical Council (2003). *Tomorrow's Doctors.* London, GMC.
General Medical Council (2006). *Good Medical Practice.* London, GMC.
Gibbs, G. (1988). In: Johns, C. (ed.) *Becoming a Reflective Practitioner.* Oxford, Blackwell Publishing.
Rinpoche, S. (1992). *The Tibetan Book of Living and Dying.* London, Rider.
Sully, P. & Dallas, J. (2005). *Essential Communication Skills for Nursing.* London, Elsevier Mosby.

Questions and answers

Q: My tutor says I do not understand the difference between reflection and description and I suppose I agree?

A: A very common misunderstanding. Any reflective process requires description of the event to some extent as a way of anchoring and capturing what happened. However, this is just stage one of the cycle and you need to go on to think about, evaluate, analyse and plan around the event. Description is just the starting point of reflection.

Q: What is the difference between the words 'reflective' and 'reflexive' as I have seen both used in books?

A: The adjective 'reflexive' describes the act of being a person who reflects, for example, *'The Dalai Lama is a reflexive thinker'* or *'Reflection is a reflexive practice'.*

Chapter 8 **Life–work balance**

> **OVERVIEW**
>
> We hope that this chapter will help you to think and plan your life at university and develop a healthy life–work balance. It includes useful ideas about time management and the organisation of study and offers some strategies for recognising and managing stress.

Why is it important?

It may seem odd to devote a whole chapter to life–work balance, but we believe that it is so important that it deserves a decent space in this book. Many students we have worked with have found it difficult to achieve a balance between their studies/work and their personal life; in fact, many of our colleagues have similar problems. It may also be a new experience for you to have to balance work and life in a self-directed way, perhaps because teachers, parents or employers have done this for you in the past. What follows are some suggestions for how this might be achieved and also some suggested issues to think about, which may be important.

You have chosen to study medicine, which is one of the most demanding university courses, and you will certainly have to work hard and devote a reasonable amount of time to it. However, the key word is **reasonable**: study should not normally become overwhelming or all consuming (except perhaps around exam times) and must be balanced against other life activities such as having fun, family/friends, sport and hobbies. Consider what you might think about a doctor who worked all the time and had no 'down time': would you think that they had a balanced view of life?

How to Succeed at Medical School: An Essential Guide to Learning, Second Edition.
Dason Evans and Jo Brown.
© 2015 John Wiley & Sons, Ltd. Published 2015 by John Wiley & Sons, Ltd.

Conversely, if you are the sort of person who has done very little study in the past (perhaps during A-Levels or a previous degree) and have relied on a good memory and cramming before exams to get through, this learning strategy will not work for long at medical school, as there is just too much to remember after a while. Again, consider what you might think about a doctor who studied very little or who spent the minimum amount of time updating his or her knowledge or skills: would you think that he or she had a balanced view of life and would you trust them with your own health?

Of course, there is no definitive rule about the amount of time you should spend studying as we are all different; however, over an average week, you should aim to be working approximately 2 hours each evening, plus about 4 hours each weekend. This sounds a lot, but is only about 12 hours per week. These hours may increase around exam times or just before hand-in dates for particular pieces of work, but in the main should not vary greatly. Some people find it easier to work in the library before going home.

> *I stay on after lectures or Case Studies and go to the library around 5.00 pm after a snack. I work until 6.30 and then go home. The rest of the evening is mine then, and I can go out, watch TV, or play computer games without feeling guilty about the work.*

Jonathan, first-year student.

As a developing health-care professional, it will be up to you to ensure that there is harmony in your life so that your mind, body and studies are in balance, and if they are not that you are able to ask for help when necessary – more about this later.

Time management

Have you noticed that we all have the same amount of time but that some people use it better than others? Can you think of someone who seems to be organised and always hits deadlines? The chances are that she/he is good at time management. Developing good time management skills can literally *set you free* to concentrate on what really matters in your life by helping to manage all the competing demands on your time in an effective way. Time management skills can be learned and are not necessarily something you are born with, and getting into good time management habits now will serve you for the rest of your life, both professionally and personally.

Ask yourself some questions:

- Do you feel overwhelmed by the amount of studying/work you have to do?
- Do you have difficulty finding lecture notes, handouts and so on, when you need them?
- Are you often behind with paying bills, doing your laundry, renewing library books and so on?
- Do you find it difficult to find a clear space to study in your room/flat?
- Do you ever find days or weeks slip by without your having achieved anything concrete?
- Do you spend lots of time making perfect notes that would win the Booker Prize, or record lectures that you never actually listen to again?
- Do you leave study/work until the last minute and then stay up all night to complete it?
- Do you have a nagging worry at the back of your mind that you have not kept up with study/work?.

If you have answered 'yes' to a few of these, then you probably need to work on your time management skills. It will take practise, but these skills quickly become embedded in everyday life until you forget about them completely.

It hit me when I had missed deadlines for three assignments, owed library fines of over £15.00 and couldn't face the mess in my room anymore that something had to be done – something had to change. I was always trying to catch up with everyone else.

Shobna, second-year student.

So, how effective are you at managing your time? Most of us are unaware of the things that take up our time and find it difficult to recall all the things we do each day. To really see what you do with your time, over the next week fill in an activity sheet for each day (Table 8.1), roughly recording the time you do things, what they are and how long they take. At the end of each day put a 'value' (high, medium or low) against each activity.

High-value activities are those that are highly essential and must be completed or progressed substantially during the day. They are activities that are directly related to your core study/work objectives and are critical to progress.

Examples: Current problem-based learning or case-based learning, all work that has an imminent deadline, preparation or research for the next day, exam or revision planning and so on.

Medium-value activities are less essential activities that it is still preferable, but less critical, to complete or progress substantially during the day. These have to be completed but the time element is less important as the impact on overall study/work objectives is less.
Examples: Deadlines for the following week/month, more long-term projects, research/preparation for medium-term work.

Low-value activities are non-essential activities that have a minor impact on your study/work objectives and can be done when time allows or given to someone else.
Examples: Rewriting lecture notes so they are neat or redrawing diagrams until they are perfect; organising the badminton club fixtures for next year; browsing the Internet with no specific search objectives; all projects with no deadlines; interruptions by text, phone, e-mail or callers.

At the end of each day, calculate the total percentage of time you have spent on each category of activity.

- For high-value activities, did you actually achieve what you set out to do?
- If not, what stopped you?
- Could you have achieved more in this category by controlling the low-value activities?
- How could you control low-value activities in the future?

There is a theory in time management called the Pareto 80/20 rule. Vilfredo Pareto was an Italian economist who suggested that 80% of income in Italy ended up in only 20% of the population's pockets! When applied in a time management context, this means that without good control, 80% of our daily activity can generate only 20% of our high-value outcomes. In other words, we can potentially spend most of our time producing very little of core importance. Look at your activity sheets (Table 8.1) for the whole week. Are there any patterns emerging? Apply the 80/20 rule. Is it true in your case?

Table 8.1 Activity sheet.

Date			
Time	Activity	Duration	Value

Procrastination

A common cause of putting off important or high value activities is something called **procrastination**, that is, putting things off that you should be doing right now. Often procrastinators cannot see the difference between urgent activities and important activities. For example:

You have been working on an assignment for the past week and are spending the afternoon writing up your research and findings ready to hand in to your tutor tomorrow. The president of the student union rings to ask you to book a room and refreshments for the meeting that is due to be held that evening in the union building. She has forgotten to do it herself and cannot get away from a lecture. You agree to do it even though you know it will take a long time and you will not finish your assignment. This is an urgent situation, but is it important? Weigh up the importance of handing in your assignment on time or having a room and refreshments for a meeting. Could you delegate this task or could you compromise by agreeing to do the room booking but not the catering?

The MindTools website has a good section on procrastination that you might like to look at as essentially we all suffer from procrastination to some extent, but some people put off important tasks so regularly that it starts to really affect their work. They may work long hours, but concentrate on the wrong tasks. They may have lots of things to do but do just one of them in great depth, leaving everything else undone. Some common causes of procrastination are:

- *feeling overwhelmed by the task you are supposed to be doing;*
- *feeling unconfident about your ability to do the task and so getting on with something you* can *do well;*
- *waiting until you feel 'in the mood' to tackle the task;*
- *fearing you will fail (or succeed) at the task;*
- *feeling you do not know how to organise the task;*
- *allowing perfectionism to get in the way ('I can't do the task perfectly, so I won't do it at all').*

(MindTools, 2006)

The way forward with procrastination is to recognise that you are doing it, work out why and then to think of personal strategies for not doing it any more. The reality is that we all have to do things we sometimes find difficult, boring or stressful and it may be helpful to make a daily 'to do' list to help you focus on what needs doing. Also, we all respond well to rewards, so perhaps part of your personal strategy could be the promise of a swim, bubble bath, night out or game of football at the end of a task?

Organisation of your week/month

By planning ahead and organising your week/month in advance, you can just concentrate on getting on and not worry that everything is not covered. Table 8.2 shows an example of a timetable designed and used by a second-year medical student.

As well as a weekly/monthly plan you will need a diary or organiser (paper or electronic) so that you can book and plan your life in advance.

Organisation of your physical environment

Trying to work in a messy or disorganised environment is always difficult. If you live in an untidy room/flat try at least to keep your desk or working

Table 8.2 Weekly timetable planner.

21–27 January	Morning	Afternoon	Evening
Monday	PBL tutorial	Lectures	4.30–6.30 study in library 8.00–9.00 yoga
Tuesday	Clinical/communication skills workshops	Work on PBL	4.00–6.00 library – prepare for GP visit 'dermatology'
Wednesday	GP visit	? swim 3.30 dentist	5.00–7.00 library work on PBL and write up reflection on GP visit
Thursday	PBL tutorial	Lectures	5.00–7.00 clinical/communication skills practice with Andre and Kim
Friday	Anatomy workshop	Lectures	Pizza and a film
Saturday	Lie in. 10.00–12.00 go over the week's lecture notes and PBL notes, file them	Washing, cooking, shopping and so on.	
Sunday	Lie in	4.00–6.00 prepare for next week	

environment clear and organised; your desk is a working machine not a place for storage. Decide on a filing system for your notes and handouts; it really does not matter which system you choose as long as it works for you. Get into the habit of reviewing your notes/handouts weekly to refresh your learning, identify any learning gaps and then file them in your system. We think that Saturday morning is a good time to do this as it signals the end of the learning week and allows a bit of unpressured time to review, plan and organise. You will revisit these notes many times over the next 4–5 years, so it will save time and energy to organise them right from the beginning. This way you get into the habit of regular review, which means that you are revising as you go along and do not have to panic near exam times.

Stress management

With a good balance of work and play in your life, there should not be too much stress to manage, particularly if you are organising your time effectively. Once you have a good time management plan going, things tend to run smoothly in the main. Stress is part of life and to some extent is good for us, helping and challenging us to perform at a high level. Stress levels fluctuate depending on what we are doing and we need to be aware of them so that we can intervene if they get too high. There are many causes of stress:

- exams
- deadlines
- presentations
- money
- relationships
- health
- family and so on.

It might be helpful to look at the physical response our bodies have to stress.

The fight/flight response

This primitive response was vital in the days when physical danger from wild animals and hostile tribes required us to either fight or run away from the danger (Figure 8.1). Of course, dangers still exist in modern society, and in order to cope with them our bodies continue to produce adrenaline to support the fight/flight response. Table 8.3 shows some of the physical changes that take place during this process.

Chapter 8

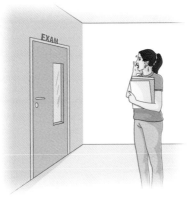

Figure 8.1   The stressed student demonstrates the fight/flight response.

Table 8.3 Physical changes taking place when stressed.

Increased activity	Decreased activity
• Pupils dilate • Circulation increases blood supply to brain, muscles and limbs • Heart beats quicker and harder: coronary arteries dilate • Blood pressure rises • Lungs take in more oxygen and carbon dioxide • Liver releases extra sugar for energy • Muscles tense for action • Sweating increases to aid heat loss blood clotting ability increases • Adrenal glands secrete adrenaline	• Digestion slows down or stops: stomach and small intestines reduce activity • Mouth goes dry: constriction of blood vessels in salivary glands • Kidney, large intestine and bladder slow down • Immune responses decrease • Sphincter muscles close to prevent urination and defecation

Stress and anxiety can trigger exactly the same fight/flight response in our bodies, but unlike being chased by a bull, there is no natural end to the response and so the adrenaline continues to circulate in our bodies triggering a physical response. The **stress/anxiety cycle** works as in Figure 8.2.

This circular motion continues unless we can break into the stress/anxiety cycle to control the physical response, and this can be done very simply by **deep breathing** and **relaxation**. By slowing down our breathing and taking in deeper breaths, we can interfere with the messages being sent to the brain and therefore control the fight/flight reflex. Look at the different physical effects stress and relaxation have on us (Table 8.4).

Table 8.4 The different physical responses of stress and relaxation.

Stress response		Relaxation response
Up	Heart rate	Down
Up	Blood pressure	Down
Up	Breathing rate	Down
Up	Muscle tension	Down
Up	Sweating	Down
Up	State of mental arousal	Down
Up	Adrenaline flow	Down

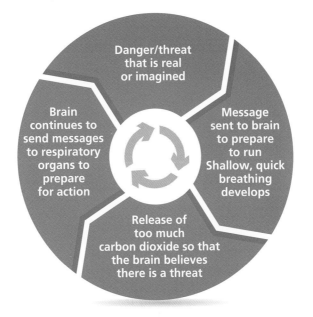

Figure 8.2 The stress/anxiety cycle.

So deep, slow breathing and periods of relaxation are important for all of us and we need to practise how to do them well. Relaxation needs to happen regularly during the day and here is a simple exercise to try.

Chapter 8

EXERCISE

- You can relax sitting in a chair, on the bus/train or lying down. It can take just 5 minutes. Make sure that you are feeling warm.
- Close your eyes and think consciously about your breathing. Take three deep in-breaths, holding them in for a few seconds before exhaling. Make sure that you empty your lungs of stale air completely.
- Think about your body systematically, starting with your feet and working up to your head and neck – consciously feel and relax each part you think about, until all of you is relaxed and heavy. Pay particular attention to your shoulders, jaw, around your eyes and forehead.
- Now in your mind, go to a beautiful or favourite place where you have felt relaxed and happy and just imagine yourself there for a few minutes.

- When you are ready, come back to where you are and become aware again of your surroundings and the sounds around you. You should feel calm, relaxed and less tense.

Interestingly, feeling relaxed and calm helps us to access memory and language skills, concentrate better, study in more depth and retain what we learn. So regular relaxation helps us with study as well as probably helping us to live a longer life!

Every time I even thought about exams I started to feel ill, my mouth and throat closed up and my stomach churned until I thought I would be sick. The student counsellor recommended I take up yoga so that I could learn to relax and control my breathing even in really stressful situations. I didn't take it seriously at first, but when I got into it I felt a bit more confident about not losing it in exams

Sam, first-year student.

Seeking help

As we mentioned earlier in this chapter, sometimes sensible balances, regular study and relaxation are not the only answers because the problems are different or deeper and you may need help from someone else. Rather than leaving things until they build up into mountains, it is better to get help sooner rather than later. It may be that you are struggling with studying or a particular topic and need extra help from a personal or specialist tutor – most tutors are really happy to help with this and can always refer you on for more specialist advice; for example, screening for particular learning difficulties such as dyslexia or dyspraxia. Most universities have specialist learning tutors to help with things such as taking good notes from lectures or writing essays – sign up to any help you can find as early as you can. In addition, many universities have good online study support and guides that you can access at a time and place that suits you.

Of course, your problems may be of a different nature and could involve drugs or alcohol, sex, money, gambling, mental health and so on. You would be in good company as many doctors suffer with the same problems. A good place to start is with the university counselling service that runs a confidential service that, if it cannot help itself, can refer you to suitable sources of help. The most important thing, though, is to be able to recognise when you do need help. These serious issues do not tend to go away by themselves, so you must resolve to take action, however hard that might be. A whole community exists to help you, not to judge you, do not be afraid to use it – be brave.

From time to time, we all need to call on our GP, Counselling Service or Student Welfare organisation, but the important issue here is that as a developing health-care professional you feel able to ask for help if life feels miserable or overwhelming for whatever reason. There is a difference between feeling anxious sometimes and feeling anxious *all* the time or between feeling sad occasionally and feeling sad *most* of the time. Medical students and doctors can lead pretty stressful lives sometimes and it is really vital to ask for help when you need it. Indeed, the mark of a competent professional is the ability to seek help when necessary.

Relaxation tips from students

'I run around the block as fast as I can to relieve stress – it works!'

'Planning and cooking a meal helps me to relax.'

'Playing computer games is my best stress buster – I have to watch this though as hours can pass unnoticed.'

'The usual stuff really, bath, bed, good book or TV.'

'I watch old episodes of Star Trek *– very relaxing.'*

'Going to the gym followed by a sauna.'

'If I wake up at night feeling stressed, I get up, write down what is worrying me and any thoughts or solutions I am thinking about and then go back to sleep. I know it is then all written down and not lost!'

'A glass of wine with friends can put things in perspective.'

Summary

We have looked at the importance of achieving a balance between life and work in this section and suggested some strategies for achieving it. We have looked at planning study and leisure and recognising procrastination as well as seeing the physical effects of stress and its management. We thought about the importance of asking for help with a wide range of problems and ended with relaxation tips from students.

- Achieving a balance between work and life is essential for the whole of professional life.
- Analyse how you use your time to see if you are effective.
- Planning and organising your time literally sets you free.
- Make a study plan each week/month and stick to it.
- Never be afraid to ask for help early.

Chapter 8

References and further reading

MindTools (2006) *Mind Tools Activity Log: Essential Skills for an Excellent Career.*
www.mindtools.com/rs/ActivityLog.

Questions and answers

Q: I already had a degree when I started at medical school and thought that I knew how much time to devote to study. But my usual two or three evenings per week are just not enough and I am only in the first year!

A: Medicine does require more hours of study than most other degrees and, because it covers such a diverse array of subjects, needs a systematic approach. 12 hours a week of well-planned study is the average, with an effective filing system to manage information and notes. As you progress on the course the nature of the study may change somewhat, particularly when you enter the clinical environment and are learning from patients.

Q: I seem to spend every evening studying, although my flatmates go out and seem to do OK in exams. Maybe I am not as bright as them?

A: This is a common concern and to a certain extent we all worry that we are not clever or good enough. Interestingly, we have almost never found this to be the case when working with students. However, anxiety can often get in the way of effective study and the key really is the quality of study rather than the quantity, although we all have individual study habits. It may be helpful to look at your flatmates' study techniques to discover how they are able to balance their lives and still be successful in exams. See Chapter 2: this discusses methods for effective study.

Q: I have to work on Saturdays and one evening during the week to support myself at medical school. The work seems to pile up and I never seem to finish.

A: It is very difficult to have a job while you are studying medicine as the course is so demanding, particularly when you reach the clinical years and may need to do on-calls or stay on to see a particular patient or procedure. You will need to develop excellent time management skills to balance all the demands and develop good study plans so that every hour of study really counts. Remember, however, that many people do need to work to support themselves and indeed many medical students have children to care for as well as studying. Be careful to ensure that you are eating and sleeping properly and have one night a week when you can completely relax.

Q: If I tell my tutor that I am struggling, won't it count against me?

A: Your tutors are involved in education because they want to help students to do well. Over the years, they have seen hundreds of struggling students and will be able to offer you good advice and support. Imagine you perform badly in an exam, if the medical school knows that you have identified a problem and that you are working to overcome it, this can only work in your favour.

Chapter 9 **Revision**

OVERVIEW

This chapter will help you plan for revision in a realistic way and will suggest some techniques that may be helpful for revising knowledge and skills. We have also collected general experiences and tips from medical students and share them here. We end as usual with commonly asked questions.

What is revision?

At a basic level, revision is a systematic way of reminding yourself of what you have learned in preparation for a written or practical exam. So much has been written in the last decade about the best ways to revise, and the most efficient techniques for committing things to memory, that choosing a personal path for revision may be confusing with so many choices available. Remember that you are already adept at passing exams because you have successfully gained GCSEs, A-levels and perhaps a degree. As you already know, revision is not rocket science, but it is a necessary part of your learning repertoire and, like anything else, revision skills can be made more effective.

We have mentioned before the importance of revising right from the beginning of the course rather than leaving things to the last minute, which can be really stressful. This way, you build your knowledge, understanding and skills gradually and systematically over time, which will increase your confidence level. If you have managed to review and organise your notes, lecture handouts, articles and so on, each week into a logical filing system, then you are already halfway there. You will have been revising as you went along and now it will simply be a matter of refreshing your understanding and perhaps getting in some practice for any practical exams.

How to Succeed at Medical School: An Essential Guide to Learning, Second Edition.
Dason Evans and Jo Brown.
© 2015 John Wiley & Sons, Ltd. Published 2015 by John Wiley & Sons, Ltd.

An important thought we would like you to hold in your mind whenever you are revising is to imagine that you are the examiner setting a question on this topic.

- What understanding would you want to test?
- What question would you ask to test it?

Having this overview always present in your mind will help you to see the knowledge and skills you have acquired from an assessment perspective and will help you to visualise the questions and tasks that you may be asked in an exam.

What kind of techniques?

So, what kind of revision techniques will work for you? Do you learn well from books? Is it better for you to discuss what you learn in a group? Are you a visual learner who enjoys diagrams or graphic representations of things? As with all learning, we are all unique and do things in different ways, but interestingly research has shown:

We remember 20% of what we read.
We remember 30% of what we hear.
We remember 40% of what we see.
We remember 50% of what we say.
We remember 60% of what we do.
We remember 90% of what we read, see, hear, say and do.

(Turner, 2007)

So, a mixture of revision methods may be useful.

Draw up a plan

It is vital to spend a few hours drawing up a comprehensive revision plan right at the start. Perhaps have one timetable for each week, decide upon the focus for that week and then break this down for each day, scheduling how long you will spend revising each topic. Remember to factor in time to eat, relax and have a period of exercise each day to counteract periods of inactivity – a long walk or a swim. Draw up revision into blocks of 1.5 hours with 30-minute gaps between to stretch your legs and get a drink. So, each revision block lasts 2 hour and you could aim to do three or four blocks for each full day, or maybe one if it is an evening session. Remember to factor in small rewards for yourself at the end of each revision period so you have something to look forward to. Factor in at least two periods each week when you will revise with others in a group. A good tip is to aim to finish your revision a week before the exam – this gives you time to revisit shaky areas and complete any fine tuning.

Providing you have made a comprehensive plan that covers the subjects to be revised and you stick to it, you can stop worrying about whether everything will be covered (Table 9.1).

Table 9.1   A sample revision timetable from a third-year student revising the heart.

Day/date	AM	PM	Evening
Monday 18 Jan	Anatomy of heart	Physiology of heart	5.00–7.00 gym and supper 7.00–9.00 draw rough anatomy, create consolidate diagrams, self-testing
Tuesday 19 Jan	Heart failure: main presentation	Heart failure: treatment and management	5.00–6.30 supper and walk 6.30–8.30 consolidation, self-testing
Wednesday 20 Jan	Myocardial infarction: main presentation	Myocardial infarction: treatment and management	6.00–7.00 supper Revising heart failure and myocardial infarction with Chris
Thursday 21 Jan	Group revision on whole topic	Revise topics identified in group revision	6.00–8.00 supper and gym Prepare for practical session tomorrow
Friday 22 Jan	Group work practising history of chest pain, examining the chest, feedback	Reflect on group practice: identify gaps and weaknesses	Epidemiology of heart disease
Saturday 23 Jan	Day off	Day off	Day off
Sunday 24 Jan	Lie in	Consolidate all topics from this week. Fine tune, finishing touches to notes. Put away files and books not needed any longer	Plan for next week's revision. Get out notes, appropriate books and so on.

Chapter 9

Three student commentaries on revision

I like to review all my (fairly extensive) notes and handouts at the end of each week and file them into module files. I then revise one module at a time in the weeks before an exam. It takes me about 4 weeks to cover each module. I don't write out special revision notes as this would be duplicating the work. I make every set of notes work for me, so it's worth getting them right from the start. I prefer revising on my own, but sometimes get together with others to practise clinical skills. I like working with other people when I don't understand something. I also like reading a wide range of text books to make sure I've got my head around everything. I revise about 5 nights a week before exams but keep weekends free for other things.

Rachel, second-year graduate student.

We set up a 'learning objectives' revision group where we look at the learning objectives for all our PBLs [problem-based learning] and clinical placements and then make sure we have covered everything, that way there are no surprises in exams. Our revision group works like a PBL group – all of us decide which aspects of a subject to find out about and we share in a group our findings. We have a scribe who records everything but I make my own notes and diagrams, which I condense into a final revision summary. I tend to start revising 8 weeks before an exam and don't do much else. I revise on most days and tend to put my life on hold.

Kris, third-year student.

Because I have two young children, it's difficult to get a routine going for revision. I try to keep my notes in order so that the course doesn't get out of control and everything is kept in a filing cabinet out of the way of the children. I often get up at 5.00 am to work as I am good in the mornings. My husband has the children all day on Saturday so I have a good stretch of time to revise in – I always go to the library though as it's quiet. I find that I can revise in a really focused way in quite small amounts of time (20 minutes) and I tend to do this throughout the day. I think having the children has taught me not to waste a minute.

Lea, first-year graduate student.

Organise your space

We talk in Chapter 8 about organising your desk or learning space. For the purposes of revision, however, we recommend a more radical reorganisation of your life! The reason for this is to minimise all distractions so that you can really concentrate on revising. So, before getting down to the work some preparation is necessary:

- clean your flat or room
- sort out and put things away
- change the bed
- organise your desk
- stock up on healthy food and snacks
- do the laundry
- tell everyone you are about to start revising
- make a 'do not disturb' notice for your door.

Think about 'known distracters': are there some things that always tend to distract you. Perhaps these are telephone calls or texts, instant messaging on your computer or switching the TV on for a second when you have a break only to find yourself sat in front of it 2 hours later. Plan how to avoid these; perhaps switch off your phone, unplug the Internet, put a towel over the TV.

If you live in a place where it is not possible to study in a quiet environment without interruption, then you will need to revise in the library or other room at your medical school. Tutors will be able to help you organise this.

During A-levels I was always able to revise everything really quickly just before exams but this didn't work for me at med school. I had to retake my second year because I failed exams on two occasions and had to learn a different way of studying for deep understanding. I think I was a late starter!

Joel, fourth-year student.

Chapter 9

Revising knowledge

An important thing for you to know is that just copying out notes from a book or handout will not help you understand or remember them. You need to interpret them and put them into your own words, perhaps by paraphrasing them or converting them into a MindMap or flow chart (Chapter 2). This is the difference between **note taking** or recording the factual content of say, a lecture and **note making**, which includes your analysis and interpretation of the information (Evans, 2004). Most exams are designed to test your understanding of a topic, not your ability to just memorise it, although there may be a small amount of information that you will need to just remember. After paraphrasing your notes, turn them over and see what you can remember and write them out again. You will now understand how useful the advice in Chapter 2 is. If you use Cornell notes or some of the other techniques that we discussed such as writing questions as you go along, this process will be much easier for you. Try revisiting your notes again in a week's time to see how much you have retained. Perhaps record your notes and try listening to them as you walk around. Pretend you are giving a lecture about this topic; what would you say and how would you organise it?

You probably already use revision cards, Post-it notes, coloured highlighter pens and mnemonics such as SOCRATES (a useful basic mnemonic when asking a patient about pain – see below). All of these are helpful tools.

- site
- onset
- character
- radiation
- associated symptoms
- timing
- exacerbating and relieving factors
- severity.

I made a batch of revision cards, which I carried about with me and looked at when I had slack time, like on the train. I find it easier to revise in short bursts rather than a long session

Alice, first-year student.

It is often said that the best way to learn something is to teach it and you may like to do this in a learning group, with everyone taking turns at teaching a topic. This works on two levels; first, it shares some of the work of the revision, but it also allows you to test your level of understanding of a topic against your peers. Are you more or less on a level with the others or are you revising a topic in too great a depth? Are you revising a good breadth or overview of a topic, but not understanding enough of the detail? Learning with others will give you a good gauge of breadth and depth.

You may like to look at past papers to get an idea of what has gone before and how questions are written and presented. Try doing some of these papers and timing yourself. Get familiar with the types of question you may be asked such as:

- extended matching questions
- multiple choice questions
- short answer questions
- best answer questions.

Being familiar with the format of the question will allow you to practise and will boost your performance. A really useful exercise is to get a group of people to sit a past paper together. Compare the results and decide upon a model answer for each question. How did others in the group tackle the question style? Chapters 10 and 11 look at common question styles and approaches to managing them in more depth.

Revising clinical and communication skills

You may already be familiar with a range of written exam formats from your previous study, but the main way that clinical and communication skills are tested at medical school is in an Objective Structured Clinical Examination (OSCE), a practical exam that may be less familiar. In an OSCE, a large room is divided into a number of 'stations', each one focused on a different task. Each station may contain a model, image, simulated patient or real patient plus an examiner and you will be asked to carry out a task in 5–10 minutes before a bell rings and you move on to the next station. The examiner will mark you on a range of items connected with the task. The great thing about OSCEs is that, although they can be nerve wracking, you get a broad range of opinion about your competency, for if there are, say, 17 stations in the OSCE, then 17 examiners assess you.

In stark contrast to revising knowledge, clinical and communication skills need to be actively revised in pairs or in a group, with **feedback**. You will probably have already covered the main skills to be revised during your course, but these must be practised, practised and practised!

We suggested earlier that just like any other sort of revision, clinical and communication skills should be practised informally on a weekly basis with your peers, although remember that revision cannot replace real experiences, but hopefully that message was clear in Chapters 3 and 4. It is also helpful if this revision is integrated. The following exercise suggests how this can be organised:

EXERCISE

An Integrated Approach to Revising Clinical and Communication Skills

- Decide as a learning group on a topic – say, asthma.
- The whole group revises the knowledge base for asthma, makes notes, diagrams, collects articles and so on.
- One member of the group writes a 'patient scenario' or role play that includes the clinical details of asthma and joins these with a relevant 'back story'

for the patient, which will include details of the patient's life and relevant psycho-social issues he or she may be experiencing.

- One person plays the 'patient' and the group take it in turns to interview the person about his or her asthma – do not forget to give each other feedback on the interview, perhaps dividing it into 'content' (the information that was gathered) and 'process' (the communication skills used to elicit the information). Use the checklist of communication skills (Chapter 4).
- The group has also looked at skills books and skills handouts on examining the chest and together you agree on a 'gold standard' for doing this and draw up a checklist.
- A group member agrees to have their chest examined and you take it in turns to examine each other using your gold standard checklist and not forgetting to give feedback.
- Do not forget to have your 'examiner's' hat on! If you were writing an OSCE station about asthma, what items would you test and what would you give marks for? We cover OSCEs in more depth in Chapter 11.

It was hard to connect all the things we had learned in lectures and PBLs [problem-based learning] to skills. I tried to learn it all from books because I'm OK at that, but in the end I realised it was about practising the skills with real people. Once I started doing that I got the hang of things.

Ryan, second-year student.

Of course, the very best way to revise clinical and communication skills is with real patients, but you may not have reached that stage of the course yet, and so working in a group with colleagues and any simulation models/equipment your medical school may have is a good substitute.

The connection between smell and memory

This connection has been well known for many years, but research at the University of Northumbria found that smelling rosemary oil 'produced a significant enhancement of performance for overall quality of memory' (Moss *et al.*, 2003) in healthy adults. This connection can be put to good use in revision. Try this:

- buy an aromatherapy oil burner and some rosemary oil (do not use rosemary oil if you are pregnant);

- burn the oil whenever you are revising, but never at any other time;
- just before going into the exam, put a few drops of rosemary oil on a tissue (never directly on to your skin) and smell it at regular intervals during the exam.

Conversely, the same research found that lavender oil significantly decreased memory and performance, so if you are finding it difficult to switch off after revision and sleep, you could try using lavender on your pillow!

General hints and tips

These have been gathered from many people and sources, but particularly from medical students who found them helpful.

- Make a 'do not disturb' notice for your door. Tell friends and family that you are revising and get their help. Stick your revision timetable on the outside of your door so that people can see what you are doing.
- Turn off your phone for regular periods when you are revising. Tell people that you are going to do this.
- Eat and drink regularly. There is a well-known connection between healthy food eaten at regular intervals and learning performance. Eat breakfast and have snacks such as bananas, sesame seeds, tuna fish, dried fruit, avocados and nuts. Drink plenty of water.
- Exercise every day to combat stress and inactivity. It will help you sleep.
- Gentle music helps some people revise and you can even buy specially designed CDs in music shops if you feel so inclined. TV, however, *never helps* – turn it off.
- Cross off each topic you revise from your revision timetable; this is deeply satisfying and charts your progress.
- Go to bed at a reasonable time and get enough sleep. Revising into the night can be counterproductive.
- Try visualising yourself entering the exam feeling calm, happy and in control. Try to imagine what the room will look like and see yourself during the exam calmly writing or performing a task in an OSCE station. Keep this positive image in your head.
- Try not to listen to what others say about an exam, particularly directly after it! People have many reasons for under or over estimating the difficulty of the exam and their performance in it. There is nothing you can do about it anyway, so just go home and do not allow yourself to be wound up.

Chapter 9

What if I fail?

Most of us fail something in our lives and miserable as that can feel, failing an exam will probably make you a better doctor. Why? Because you will develop strategies to overcome the failure and pass re-take exams, and you will have gained valuable experience and insight into what it feels like to fail, which in turn will develop your empathic skills.

Failing an exam is not the end of the world, even if it feels like it at the time, and most medical schools will be able to offer you some help and support in preparing for a re-take exam or repeating part of the course. Get as much feedback as you can about why you have failed so that you can identify your strengths and weaknesses, get together with any others who have also failed to develop a plan and form a learning group to prepare for what comes next.

Try talking to students in the years above you about their revision techniques and tips; often they will have developed sophisticated strategies and there is never any point reinventing the wheel! Conversely though, no one strategy fits everyone and you will need to design revision around your own strengths and weaknesses and learning style.

Summary

In this section, we have looked at what revision is and what is not. We have highlighted the differences between revising knowledge and skills and looked at the connection between smell and memory. We have highlighted the practical implications of drawing up a good revision plan and managing your revision space and have seen examples of revision strategies from three students and some suggestions for integrated revision in a group.

- View the subject you are revising from an examiner perspective.
- Exams test understanding and not memory.
- Revise from the beginning of the course.
- Make a good revision plan and stick to it.
- People revise in a variety of effective ways.
- Spend some time revising in a group.

References and further reading

Evans, M. (2004). *How To Pass Exams Every Time*. Oxford, How To Books Ltd.

Moss, M., Cook, J., Wesnes, K., Duckett, P. *et al.* (2003). Aromas of rosemary and lavender essential oils differentially affect cognition and mood in healthy adults. *International Journal of Neuroscience, 113*, 15–38.

Turner, L.K. (2007). *Revision Techniques, Business Studies*. Wood Green, London, Woodside High School.

Questions and answers

Q: I seem to spend hours revising but cannot remember anything in the exam.

A: A common problem that may be due to poor revision technique. You may spend hours revising, but is it quality revision? Have you made a timetable, allocated topics to blocks of time, paraphrased your notes and shared revision with a group? It is really about the quality of the revision and not the quantity. Beginning your revision in good time will also increase your confidence because you will know you have everything covered.

Q: I seem to panic just before going into an exam.

A: Exams can be very stressful and most people feel a bit panicky at the start. Remember that this panic will cause a 'fight or flight' reaction. Go through the breathing and relaxation techniques suggested in Chapter 8 and think about a more long-term solution such as yoga. If this becomes a really big problem for you, then you need to seek help from your counselling service who may be able to help you develop individual strategies to combat your panic.

Q: I lost a load of my revision notes on the bus.

A: This bad luck can be turned into a really good revision tool! Ask to borrow other people's notes, look at the books to check the content, paraphrase them into something that makes sense to you. Compare revision notes for depth and breadth, present what you have learned in a group. By doing all of this, you are actively revising and may even revise more effectively this way!

Q: I never know how soon to start revising before an exam.

A: I hope that we have convinced you that revision is something you should be doing as you go along every week and that the last few weeks before an exam should be a time for fine-tuning and consolidation, as you will not be able to cram a year of learning into 5 weeks! A few weeks before the exam, draw up a revision timetable so that you can review and remind yourself of what you have learned. Leave plenty of time so things are not rushed and there is time to cover things in enough detail.

Chapter 9

Chapter 10 **Exam technique: general rules**

OVERVIEW

This chapter provides an overview of the general rules for any exam. Many of these are simple and yet we know from many students that they can be neglected. You will read most of this chapter quickly, and we suspect that it will make a lot of sense. You might want to read it again a week or two before you sit your first set of exams, perhaps subsequent sets of exams too.

In Chapter 11, we shall try and apply these general principles to the specific exams that you are likely to come across in your time at medical school.

Introduction

This chapter brings bad news and good news. The bad news is that contrary to popular belief, cunning exam technique will not allow you to pass exams at medical school without doing any work. The good news, however, is that appropriate exam technique will help you demonstrate what you know to your advantage.

Preparing for the exam

Knowing the format and rules of the exam

Students who struggle often tell us: 'I didn't know what to expect from the exam'. It might seem obvious, but you should invest some time **finding out about the exam**, including its structure and format. How many questions, how much time and what sort of questions will there be? All this information is crucial to your preparation. There will be formal information, such as exam

How to Succeed at Medical School: An Essential Guide to Learning, Second Edition.
Dason Evans and Jo Brown.
© 2015 John Wiley & Sons, Ltd. Published 2015 by John Wiley & Sons, Ltd.

briefings and written information, but do not forget the informal information, including impressions from students in the year above: 'There was much more anatomy than I was expecting' or 'I didn't realise that the questions would expect us to explain pathology in terms of what we knew of anatomy and physiology' will be invaluable to you.

One word of warning though, remember that these are rather subjective judgements. At one institution we know, performance in the third-year exams would oscillate: one year many students would fail the clinical exam and few the written; these students would then pass on the message that the clinical exam was really hard and 'no-one ever failed the written' and the following year students would come well prepared for the clinicals, but poorly prepared for the writtens. This caused a rather predictable 2-year cycle. You might, therefore, try and speak to students in several years above you and try and build a consensus on their advice. Think about useful questions that you could ask, such as:

- What exactly happened in the exam?
- What was different from what you expected?
- If you were doing the exam again, what would you do differently in your preparation?

If you know the format of the exam, you can practise some **mock exams**. Perhaps you will use past papers, questions from books or the Internet or even write your own (see our previous discussions about writing questions as you study in Chapter 2). As we discussed in Chapter 9, perform under exam conditions and especially under exam timings. Use these practice papers as a chance to practise technique and also as a diagnostic tool. If you get a question wrong, **do not** just memorise the right answer, but rather go back and revise that area again. Imagine that you get a question on one of the treatments of diabetes wrong; this probably means that you need to look at all the treatments of diabetes again, perhaps even that you need to ensure that you understand the whole of diabetes.

Extenuating circumstances

Every institution has an **extenuating circumstances** policy. You may not wish to think about this, but imagine that something terrible happens to you around the time of an exam: perhaps a family member falls ill or water starts pouring into your flat and you have to camp out on a friend's floor. In these cases, your institution might take these circumstances into account when looking at your results. Examples might include (different for each institution):

- If you do not turn up for an exam, this is usually counted as a fail, reducing the number of further attempts that you can have at this exam and placing a bit of a black mark on your record. If you have good reason, the exam board might agree to make the next sitting of the exam that you do count as a 'first sit'.
- If something terrible has happened to you around the time of the exam, and your result comes out at just a very little below the pass mark, the exam board might look at your extenuating circumstances and agree that they prevented you from demonstrating your true level on the day of the exam.

True to form, when things go wrong, the last thing you will want to do is try and find out the regulations and paperwork for extenuating circumstances. Get these papers together well before the exam and keep them somewhere safe; hopefully you will not need them, but you or a friend might be grateful for your preparation one day.

While talking about extenuating circumstances, we ought to also highlight a few points. First, exam boards really are not impressed with frivolous claims: if your hamster died 2 months before the exam, they are really unlikely to want to hear about it. They only want to know if there is a valid reason that your performance *on the day* did not reflect your knowledge and skills. Similarly, if you have a long-standing problem that has affected your work, perhaps your recurrent admissions to hospital with asthma and chest infections has meant that you missed most of the teaching this year and then you fail the exam, they might surmise that you did not have the knowledge and skills required for you to pass the exam because of all the time you lost and so you should, indeed, have failed. If you were in A&E all night the night before the exam with an asthma attack and wheezed your way through the exam after a sleepless night, they might, instead, surmise that it would be reasonable for your mark to be a little higher.

The university learning support unit thought that I might have dyslexia, they referred me to an educational psychologist who confirmed it and wrote a report for the exams office. I now have extra time in written exams and feel far less stressed.

Jamie, second-year medical student.

Clearly, any claim you make will need to be honest and you will need to be able to provide written evidence to back up your claim. Whatever happens, do not lie. If things are going wrong for you in the lead up to the exams, just as at any other time, do not forget that the school would rather know about it sooner than later and that people are in place to help and support you (Chapter 8). Most extenuating circumstances policies only work if you make the school aware of your difficulties before the exam, and *never* after the results are out.

Rather than an 'extenuating circumstances policy', some Medical Schools now have a 'fit-to-sit' policy that states that if you sit an exam, in doing so you are declaring yourself fit to do so. In these institutions proof of extenuating circumstances may be able to strike that attempt of the exam (that you did not sit) from the record, rather than count it as a fail. Hopefully this makes the clear point that you must know your institution's regulations.

Learning from the past

The final thing to consider before the exam is your **previous experience**. How have previous exams gone? Where are your strengths and weaknesses? If you often get too nervous before an exam, you should plan months in advance what you can do about this (see the next section and Chapter 8). Similarly if you find a certain format of exam particularly challenging, then you should actively plan how to address this before the exams. Some tips in the following sections might help, as will various courses that your school will run. Students who say 'it's funny, but I never do well in multiple choice exams' do not get much sympathy!

Dealing with nerves

Everyone gets nervous before an exam. This is normal, and indeed a bit of adrenaline probably helps you perform better. If you have been following the advice in this book, then you should have learnt the content of the course and revised it as you have gone along, using deep techniques that ensured understanding and effective recall (Chapter 2), you will have revised well (Chapter 9), and you can relax in the knowledge that you are well prepared.

Of course, some people get very nervous at exam time, and in addition to the advice that we gave in Chapter 9 (revision) there are some simple tips to follow on the day.

- **Be early for the exam** – the last thing you want to feel on the day is the panic that you might not make it in time for the exam. Aim to arrive at least half an hour (more if you are travelling a distance to get there) before the start of the exam.
- **Speak only to people who will make you feel good about the exam** – this advice from Stella Cottrell (2006) is important. Louise's advice below gives a good example of learning from experience.

I failed my first year exams because I was too nervous – I turned up and stood outside the exam hall with all my friends, and listening to them talk about all the things that they had learned made me panic, and in the exam all I could do was think that I hadn't prepared enough, rather than the questions in front of me.

Every exam I have taken since then, I have arrived early but waited quietly in a nearby seminar room or café, glancing through my notes and practising yoga breathing, and gone through to the exam on time.

I haven't failed an exam since.

Louise, newly-qualified doctor.

- **Sometimes people panic in the exam** – there are always one or two students who look at the first question and feel panic. Some run out of the exam hall. This is simple stage fright, it happens every time an actor steps onto stage, every time a lecturer steps into the lecture theatre and every time a student turns over the exam paper. If this happens badly to you, badly enough for you to get up and try and run out, do not worry, it has happened many times before and the invigilators should be well prepared. Make sure that an invigilator goes with you and let them talk to you. Halfway through their friendly pep-talk to you, you are likely to interrupt them and ask if you can go back into the exam. When you look again at the questions, you will realise that some do not look so bad!

During the exam

Read the instructions for the exam

How many questions should you answer, in what time? You should have found out this information well in advance and practised timings in the mock exams that you sat, but check that nothing has changed. Watch out for easy errors that you could make. Instructions such as 'Answer three questions from section A, four questions from section B and one question from section C' are a recipe for disaster. Write in big letters in section A 'THREE QUESTIONS', in section B 'FOUR QUESTIONS' and section C 'ONE QUESTION' right at the start, so that in the heat of the exam you do not get thrown.

Read the question

This might seem like a patronising point, but as examiners we have seen hundreds of examples of students not reading the question and so losing out on demonstrating what they know. Some examples are shown in Table 10.1.

The key way of ensuring that you read the question is to carry a pen with you and draw a box around, underline or otherwise highlight each of the key words or phrases (Chapter 2) in the question; examples are listed in Table 10.2. One word of warning, you may not be allowed to write on the question sheet;

Table 10.1 Examples of students not reading the questions properly.

Q1 The following are classical features of left heart failure (multiple choice question)	Student reads 'right' heart failure and gets each answer wrong
Q2 Please teach this patient how to use these inhalers and explain how each one works (OSCE question)	Student just teaches how to use the inhaler and misses out on half the marks
Q3 List four causes of clubbing, each originating from pathology in a different organ (short answer question)	Student lists only three causes or student lists four causes originating from lung disease only
Q4 Doctors make populations less healthy – discuss (essay question)	Student only gives one point of view (so does not 'discuss'). Student focuses on health policy (and not 'doctors'). Student focuses on treatment of disease ('health' does not only refer to the absence of disease)
Q5 This patient complains of intermittent yellowing of the skin, please conduct an abdominal examination and present your findings to the examiner – you have 5 minutes (clinical examination/OSCE question)	Student spends 4 minutes trying to take a history from the patient (no marks), only manages a very brief examination and does not have time to present

Table 10.2 Examples of highlighting key points in exam questions.

Q1 The following are *classical features* of *left* heart failure

Q2 Please *teach* this patient how to use these inhalers and *explain* how each one works

Q3 List *four* causes of *clubbing*, each originating from pathology in a *different organ*

Q4 *Doctors* make *populations* less *healthy – discuss*

Q5 This patient complains of intermittent yellowing of the skin, please conduct an *abdominal examination* and *present your findings* to the examiner – you have 5 minutes

Chapter 10

for example, in a clinical exam where other students will be looking at the same question sheet. Our advice remains the same but rather than actually write on the question, simply imagine that you are doing so – which words or phrases *would* you highlight?

Plan your answer

Depending on the sort of exam that you are sitting, you may have more or less time to plan your answer. If you are answering essay questions, then you might have a good deal of time to plan. Short answer questions might warrant a minute of planning and in clinical examinations you might have only a few moments for planning (e.g. when introducing yourself and gaining consent in an Objective Structured Clinical Examination (OSCE) you might add in the plan- '. . . I would like to run through how to use these inhalers and also cover how each one works . . . Is that OK with you? . . .') We will cover planning in more depth when talking about each exam format, but the key point is that you should avoid leaping into an answer without having some idea how you will go about that answer.

Manage your time carefully

One of the commonest errors in exams is running out of time and so not answering every question. You must be rigorous with your timing. For multiple choice questions, missing out 10% of the questions because you run out of time will drop your final mark by up to 10%. Not answering one of four essay questions will drop your final mark by 25%; the maths is easy, but people still do it. Two problems lead to students not finishing in time. One is planning: we would recommend that you write key time points into different parts of the question paper (we have called these '**time-posts**'), and that you practise your timing in mock exams. The second reason is a strong desire to write a perfect answer. Look at the following example: most marks (easy marks) are gained in the first half or two-thirds of the time spent on each question, after that additional marks become increasingly more costly (in terms of time) to gain.

Planning your time

Imagine that you have 10 minutes to write about the clinical presentation of myocardial infarction (a heart attack), which will give you 10 points. This is one of 10 short answer questions that you have to answer.

You might plan to answer the question under the headings of 'classical presentation' and 'non-classical presentation'. Within 5 minutes you write about classical presentations and gain six easy marks. Having written all the obvious things, gaining additional marks starts to take more time. Over the next 2 minutes you gain a further mark and then over the last 3 minutes you get one more mark.

In 10 minutes, you have scored 8/10 and it is time to move on. You could stay on this question, wracking your brain, but it might take another 5 minutes to get up to 9/10, by which time you have lost out on the opportunity of getting the six 'easy' marks on the next question.

A score of 8/10 on all 10 questions gives 80% and 9/10 on seven questions and 0/10 on the remaining three (ran out of time) gives 63%.

You have to be tough with yourself on the timing, when you are out of time for that question move on. You can always come back to it at the end if you have time. Note that, even if you do not know much about the answer to a question, you are better off making a stab at it and getting maybe half marks for that question than spending that time on a question that you know more about and getting perhaps one additional mark. *Answer all the questions that you are supposed to answer.*

After the exam

Many students loiter outside the exam hall talking about the questions. This helps some students let off steam, but for others, watching a colleague look through the books and punch the air saying 'Yes, another one I got right!' every minute or so can be irritating at best and disastrous for self-confidence for the next exam at worst. So you might want to walk away and treat yourself to something nice.

At some point on the same day of the exam, find some time to sit down and write some reflections – what went well, what helped, what did not go so well and what led up to this. From these reflections, write down a plan for preparing for the next exams and stick to it. It might be something simple like bringing an extra pencil or something as insightful as Louise's example mentioned earlier. You might want to share your ideas with other students in your study group. They might have some additional ideas that would be useful to you and yours might well be useful to them. The key message here is to learn from experience and to continue to improve.

Messages from the other side

We, the authors, as examiners, have four key messages to share with you. Believe them or not (and you will not believe them all), they remain true and relevant. They relate to the purpose of the assessment, the motivations of the examiners, having some empathy for the examiners and the noble art of question spotting.

Know why you are being assessed

Assessment has various purposes. These include acting as a hurdle (to ensure that you know enough to progress into the second year or that you are skilled, knowledgeable and safe enough to graduate as a doctor), to provide you with feedback (e.g. to help your academic writing skills develop or to highlight your weaker areas to you) and to provide feedback on the course (if three-quarters of the year do not know the names of the valves of the heart, there is probably something wrong with the course rather than the students).

Chapter 10

Students often lose the focus of knowing why they are being assessed. Most institutions' final exams are focused on ensuring that graduates are knowledgeable enough, skilled enough and safe enough to become first-year junior doctors. Some students think that *finals* are *much more* and try and study up to some hyper-advanced level and as a result might have trouble covering all the bases. More worryingly, some students think that finals are *much less*, and their focus is just on finding a 'trick' to passing the exam, to 'performing' well on the day, to learn just the topics that they think will come up. These students, usually not ready to be doctors, tend to do badly. We have discussed depth versus breadth in your studying elsewhere in this book (Chapter 2), knowing the purpose of the assessment will guide you in your judgement of how to decide how deep to go in your preparation for an exam.

Examiners are out to help

Contrary to popular belief, examiners are really, honestly *not* out to get you. A huge amount of effort is put into trying to make the exam as fair as possible, trying to spot every single way that a student might get the wrong end of the stick and working out ways to prevent this from happening. If a question just asks you to list four causes of something, there really will be no marks for a fifth cause and the examiners really do not want you to list all the treatments too. There are really no hidden messages and things to read between the lines.

The examiners truly want you to pass, to do well. They will try hard to get the best out of you in order to help you get the best possible marks. Ironically, this might include asking you difficult, sometimes impossible questions to see how you go about trying to answer them. You might find these challenging questions 'unfair' but give them your best shot, you might be surprised by the results.

Transference

Transference is a term from clinical psychology whereby a patient assumes that their therapist or doctor is feeling the same as them at a given time. You will be aware of this from your own life. Whenever you have been embarrassed, you probably assumed that the rest of the world was embarrassed too. Buying condoms for the first time from a chemist or supermarket is a good example. You are likely to feel that everyone is looking at you and that the person behind the till is thinking something about you, whereas, of course, although this might be the first time you have ever bought condoms, this is the ten-thousandth time that they have sold them, and they are unlikely to even be consciously aware of the fact.

The same happens in exams: students enter the exam room very anxious and in a hypersensitive state of awareness. For these students, everything is directed at them. An examiner yawns and this is a personal message aimed at the student (in reality, the examiner was up all night with a new baby and has just sat through 99 other students performing the same skill, over and over again, on a hot summer's day). Because of this transference, many students can be thrown in the exam, their anxiety levels spiralling out of control.

The key to control is recognition. If you know that the feeling in your gut is just transference and that everyone around you is as anxious as you are, then you can smile and let it pass. If ever you get the chance to be an examiner yourself, even for a mock exam, jump at the chance. Understanding the examiner's perspective is hugely valuable.

> *My medical school put on a mock OSCE where I played the candidate, and in the second half I was an examiner. I didn't expect it, but I learnt much more from being an examiner.*

Tuan, fourth-year medical student.

Examiners are only human too

Examining is often tediously boring. Marking essay after essay on the same topic, trying to spot key points in short answer question after short answer question or listening to 150 students in a day ask a simulated patient how much alcohol he or she drinks and whether he or she has ever thought of cutting down, just is not fun. If you know this and if you can put yourself in the examiners' shoes, then you can make their life easier and in doing so help them to spot the marks that you deserve.

Make sure that your answers are easy to follow. If your handwriting is terrible, work on improving it and write key points in capitals so that they stand out. Consider two responses to the following short-answer question.

Q6 Describe the initial clinical presentations of myocardial infarction (a heart attack), (10 points)

RESPONSE 1> Myocardial infarction can present with chest pain, not relieved by glyceryl trinitrate. Sometimes, there might be no pain. Patients might vomit and often look generally unwell. The pain may or may not be present and may be confused with indigestion. It is classically central and radiates to the left arm or chin, and may be described as crushing, although sometimes there might be no pain. History gained from the patient or their relatives might be suggestive of an increase in cardiovascular risk factors and sometimes blood tests would have revealed a raised cholesterol in the past or raised blood pressure or angina. Blood pressure at the time of myocardial infarction might be high or low or normal. Myocardial infarctions that do not present might present late with fever or sometimes heart failure

RESPONSE 2>
CLASSICAL PRESENTATION:
Symptoms

- Chest pain – classically CRUSHING, CENTRAL, may RADIATE to left arm or chin. NOT RELIEVED by nitrates or rest
- Associated symptoms – SWEATING, NAUSEA, VOMITING, collapse, breathlessness
- Past history – may have past history of ANGINA or OTHER CARDIOVASCULAR RISK FACTORS (cholesterol, raised blood pressure, arterial disease)

Signs

- May look GENERALLY UNWELL – sweaty, tachycardia, in pain
- BLOOD PRESSURE up or down or normal
- May present with CARDIAC ARREST

ATYPICAL PRESENTATIONS

- Atypical chest pain (indigestion)
- FEVER ± HEART FAILURE about 12 hours post MI
- CARDIAC ARREST
- ASYMPTOMATIC MYOCARDIAL INFARCTION – found at screening at some later date

---

Imagine that you are marking both these answers and that you have a marking scheme that lists all the key words that would earn the candidate a mark (and will probably rather look like response 2). The candidate who gave this response, therefore, has made your life easy, and it is simple to tick each key point. It is much harder to spot the marks in the script labelled response 1>.

Question spotting and blueprinting

As a student, one of the authors spent many hours looking through past papers for recurring themes and patterns, making charts and graphs and trying to second-guess the examiners. If a topic tended to come up every other year and did not come up last year, it would surely come up this year. This is a common pastime among medical students, with days or weeks wasted trying to predict the future. Some graduate and go on to play the stock market, producing similar graphs of share prices, but most of us learned sooner or later that it was pointless!

When setting the content of an exam, examiners go through a process called blueprinting. In this process, they look at the content of the curriculum and ensure that the exam (or exams) samples a wide range of the curriculum that is expected to have been covered by this stage of your training. The blueprint puts a little more weight on important things, so more questions will fall into this category, but the blueprint ensures that everything that should have been covered could be covered in the exam. This is why it is important for you to think about **the purpose of the exam**: this will give you a clue as to the likely content.

Here is the bad news. In addition to looking to the curriculum to build the blueprint of the exam, they also tend to look to the blueprints of the same exam in previous years; they will *know* if a certain question tends to come up every other year, and they will *know that the students know*. To avoid alternate years of students not learning the topic, they might decide to drop it in to an 'unexpected' year or leave it out for a couple of years.

Really dedicated examiners will even turn to the blueprints of the other exams that you have sat, and will be sitting in the future, to ensure that there is a really good spread of topics, with important things (diabetes, heart attacks etc.) coming up quite a few times and rarer/less important things covered less often, but still making an outing from time to time.

If you wish, therefore, to guess the content of the exam, ensure that you know the purpose of the exam and the level expected. From this, you will be able to list the important and common topics that are likely to come up – you need to know these well – and also the less common topics that might come up – you will need to know enough about these to be 'good enough' at the level of the exam. Making predictions any more specific than this is just a waste of time that you could be spending studying.

Chapter 10

Chapter 11 **Exam technique: specific examples**

OVERVIEW

This chapter first describes the range of assessments used in medical education and then applies the general rules covered in Chapter 10 to specific examples. Note that although there are some very good general books available on exam technique in higher education (see *References and Further Reading*), it is hard to find any that provide useful advice on the range of assessments used specifically in medical courses. Each medical school seems to add its own flavour to its assessments, so supplement these rather generic pages with discussions with the other students in your year, those in the years above, any past papers in the library and any friendly faculty members that you come across.

Introduction

It would be rather dull to punctuate each paragraph with a disclaimer, so here is one reminder that good exam technique helps you to effectively demonstrate what you know/can do. It does not, in any way, replace the fact that you need to have learnt the content first! You must also remember from the first section of Chapter 10 that you should make every effort to find out the exact format of the exams at your school. As you will read in the following sections, everyone has their own specific variations based on common themes.

How to Succeed at Medical School: An Essential Guide to Learning, Second Edition.
Dason Evans and Jo Brown.
© 2015 John Wiley & Sons, Ltd. Published 2015 by John Wiley & Sons, Ltd.

Types of exams

Multiple-choice exams

By multiple-choice exams, we refer to any assessment when you are asked to choose between different options in order to demonstrate that you know something. These are popular exams, not least because they are easy to mark using automatic systems, such as optical readers (you mark on a standardised answer sheet, in pencil and a computer scanner reads your answers and calculates your marks, along with a whole lot of exam statistics, in seconds) and even direct-entry exams where you interact with a computer (removing the need for someone to stand over a computer scanner cursing every time it gets jammed). Examples of different multiple-choice formats are described below.

True/false items
Each item is independently marked as either true or false.

These are generally less popular in medical education as they tend to test regurgitation of simple facts rather than understanding and tend not to allow for the fact that there is often not a single answer. Some schools still use them quite a lot.

Example true–false multiple-choice question

Q7 With regard to diabetes:

A. Insulin resistance is commoner in type 2 (late onset) than type 1 diabetes (T)

B. A single fasting blood glucose of greater than 5.0 is diagnostic (F)

C. Women who develop diabetes in pregnancy are more likely to develop diabetes in later life (T)

Best of five
In these questions, you are asked to choose from a list of five items and choose the one that is *most true* or *most relevant* to the lead in (or 'stem') of the question. This allows for uncertainty and some degree of judgement. Q8 gives an example of how some simple true/false questions can be converted into a best-of-five format (here, best of three). In Q9, both items B and C might be true but B is less clear, more debatable than C, so the correct answer is C.

Example 'best of five' format

Q8 With regard to diabetes, which of the following statements is TRUE?

A. Insulin resistance is commoner in type 1 (early-onset) diabetes than type 2

B. A single fasting blood glucose of greater than 5.0 is diagnostic

C. Women who develop diabetes in pregnancy are more likely to develop diabetes in later life (CORRECT)

Chapter 11

Q9 With regard to study skills, which of the following statements is most true?
A: Drawing a MindMap is only possible if you have A3 paper
B: The Cornell method is best used in lectures
C: It takes about 3 months to learn a new study skill effectively (CORRECT)
D: Study skills tend to make little difference to performance
E: Copying out chunks of text from a textbook is an active learning
technique

Extended matching questions (EMQs)
This format of questions is becoming rather common in medical education. Each question (stem) has a general topic, followed by a range of possible answers. The student is then presented with a number of question items (often in the form of a scenario) and he or she needs to select one (or sometimes more than one) answer for each item from the list of possible answers.

Example of extended matching questions

A	True/false multiple-choice		G	Objective structured clinical examination
B	Best of five		H	Viva voce examination
C	Extended matching questions		I	Portfolio-based assessment
D	Short answer questions		J	Computer-marked assessment
E	Essay questions in an examination		K	Blood test
F	Non-timed essay questions			

Each of the following descriptions relates to a different form of assessment. Choose the **single most appropriate answer** from the aforementioned list.

Q10 A student who graduated in the 1980s sat this knowledge-based exam and had to select whether each of 600 items relating to basic and clinical sciences were true or not.

Q11 A medical school decides to replace the traditional assessments in the final year with this method that requires students to collect evidence from a wide range of sources to demonstrate that they have the required attributes to graduate.

This format allows examiners to ask some reasonably probing questions to try and assess **understanding** rather than just knowledge and even some **problem-solving skills**.

The situational judgement test

Changes in medical education unfortunately tend to occur in quite large leaps rather than small gentle steps. At the time of writing this second edition, the current big leap occurring is the introduction of a 'new' form of assessment called the situational judgement test (SJT). It is actually not new at all and has been around in other walks of life for many years, perhaps since the late 1800s or perhaps the mid-1900s depending on what source you read. It has been nicely demonstrated that if they are constructed well, the assessments can have both validity (measures what it is supposed to measure) and reliability (score due to ability rather than 'noise'). They were introduced as an assessment for final-year medical students in the academic year 2012–2013, with the intention that the score on the SJT, combined with a measure of academic performance, would result in some kind of a ranking that would enable a more fair allocation of the first job as a junior doctor. It was an entirely new form of assessment for most of the students sitting it, it is fair to say that it did not go down too well, and as a method of assessment causes much stress. The concept behind SJTs is a good one it is already being adopted in other branches of medical education. We have included a section later in this chapter to try and deal with some of the myths around SJT and give some gentle, sensible advice on how to approach them.

SJTs are a useful tool for assessing people's choices in situations where the best option is not always clear. Good ones go through a rigorous creation and piloting programme that is nicely summarised in the 'monograph' listed under *Further reading*. This is important to remember, because they are really hard to write well, and a lot of the revision books with mock SJTs in them were written rather quickly and have variable quality questions in them. Do not let the quality, or lack of clarity, of some of these mock questions put you off the national assessment. The same goes for the examples that we have made up here! There is a sample paper of genuine questions that you can do online and get detailed, useful feedback; it can be found on the foundation programme website listed under further reading.

There are lots of different types of SJT, but currently only two forms are used in foundation-year application: questions requiring ranking of a number of answers and questions requiring choosing three best answers (which, confusingly, they call 'multiple-choice'). In the ranking questions, these are marked out of a possible maximum mark of 20. You get four marks for each item, which is ranked in the right place (e.g. you rank the best answer first), three

Chapter 11

marks for each item, which is one place off (e.g. you rank the best answer as second), two marks for each item two places off (you rank the middle answer last), one mark for three places off (you rank the second best answer last) and no marks for more than three places off. For the 'best three answer' questions, there is a maximum of 12 marks, 4 for each correct answer. If you choose more than three items, you score zero.

Example

You are an FY1 (Foundation Year 1, your first year as a doctor) on a very busy general medical ward. Over the last few days, you have developed a cough and wheeze and have started to get some mild fevers. You suspect that you are developing a chest infection and you do not want to get ill and have to go off sick, as that would really leave your colleagues with an exceptionally high workload.

Please rank the following options in order of most appropriate to least appropriate.

A Take some appropriate antibiotics from the medication trolley, as you noticed that there were plenty left from a patient who has now gone home.

B Ask a colleague who is an FY2 to write you a private prescription for some antibiotics.

C Telephone your GP, explain the situation and ask for an urgent appointment. Let your consultant know that you will need to take a few hours off to see your GP.

D Ask one of the consultant chest physicians to see you at the end of their clinic, off the record.

E Go down and queue in A&E at the end of your shift.

Example

You are an FY1 working on a surgical ward. One of you colleagues is currently off sick and the workload is very busy. It is Monday morning and you have spent all the weekend with diarrhoea and vomiting, unable to keep anything down. You have not eaten anything unusual and suspect that you had caught a bug, there is a lot of gastroenteritis around at the moment. This morning you feel drained but well enough for work, you have had breakfast and kept it down. You are keen to go in as you know it will be horrible for your colleagues if you do not.

Choose the THREE most appropriate actions to take in this situation.

A Go into work, making sure that you wash your hands frequently.

B Go into work, and try to swap so that you assist in the operating theatre, wearing a mask and gloves.

C Stay home, rest and catch up on reading the journals.

D Ask for an emergency appointment to see your GP today.

E Telephone your consultant or senior member of the team to tell them that you are sick.

F Telephone your educational supervisor to tell them that you are sick.

G Telephone human resources and tell them you are sick today.

H Telephone the other FY1s and ask if they can manage without you.

Written exams

Essays

Essays will be familiar to all students. At medical school, you will be required to write some essays, certainly as assignments within coursework, and still in some schools as part of formal exams. Essays are tiresome to mark and can be challenging to mark fairly. As a result, they seem to feature less often within medical school assessments and when they do, students can feel unprepared. We have not included a section on essays in this chapter, but have included some information on essays and academic writing in Chapter 6.

Short answer questions

These questions ask students to write, in free text, what they know about a subject. Questions are usually structured and more focused, and answers are usually given in note form as shown in the example in Chapter 10. Some institutions give single questions (e.g. Q12), others break a question down into sub-parts to help structure the answer (Q13). The marking scheme is usually very apparent and candidates usually write their answers directly on the question sheet, including any rough working.

Q12 Describe the initial clinical presentations of myocardial infarction (a heart attack) (10 points)

Q13 Describe the classical acute symptoms of a myocardial infarction (4 marks)

Describe the key findings likely on examination of a patient suffering from a myocardial infarction (3 marks)

List the principal initial investigations required to confirm a myocardial infarction (3 marks)

Clinical exams

If you are to graduate as a doctor, clearly it is important that you will be able to demonstrate that you can apply your knowledge and skills directly with patients. Traditionally, this was tested through **long and short cases**: long cases where you saw one or two patients, took their history, examined them and tried to work out what was going on before presenting your findings to the examiners and answering questions, and short cases where the examiners would take you to see 'bits' of patients to see if you could spot what was going on. On one session, you might see three different sorts of arthritis of the hand, listen to a couple of different heart murmurs and feel a lump in someone's abdomen, all with barely time to even introduce yourself to the patients who were attached to these various clinical signs.

These exams had their strengths, but unfortunately two students might have a very different experience, with one perhaps having 'easier' patients than another. Long and short cases have largely (but not completely) been replaced with Objective Structured Clinical Examinations (OSCEs). Imagine a big hall, with 24 booths around the walls – six on each side. Each booth tests a different skill. In booth or 'station' 1, a student might be expected to take blood from a rubber arm, in station 2 a student might be expected to ask a patient about their chest pain in order to come to a diagnosis, in station 3 perhaps students examine a patient's arthritic hands and so forth. Twenty-four students stand there, one in each station, and spend a specified time in each one (let us say 5 minutes) and at the 5-minute bell each student moves on to the next station – apart from the student at station 24, who moves to station 1. After 120 minutes, every student has done every station and the exam is over. Every student has had the same experience.

Add some variations in timing (perhaps some stations last 10 minutes and some last 5 minutes), in design (perhaps it is made up of two 12-station exams held at different times, include some 'rest' stations where students can sit and worry) and in location (perhaps it is not in one big hall but instead students move in and out of pokey offices and tutorial rooms desperately looking for the way to the next station) and you have an OSCE. Fair because every student gets the same experience, safe because a wide range of skills are tested so unsafe students do not slip through unspotted, incredibly dull for the examiners and either quite fun or absolute torture for the students, depending on their perspective. Love them or hate them, OSCEs remain the gold-standard assessment of clinical competence and look set to remain so for a while yet.

Clearly, OSCEs are not very realistic and as a response to calls for assessments that truly assess what people can and do in the real life care of patients, various work-based assessments have been proposed. The most widely used in the United Kingdom is the **Mini Clinical Evaluation Exercise**

(**Mini CEX**, pronounced mini C-E-X). There are a multitude of variations in this theme, but simply put the candidate performs some kind of task, usually with a patient, and is observed and marked by a senior using a semi-structured *pro forma*. Over the months and years, they are observed by many different people while performing many different clinical tasks with many different patients and an overall picture or judgement can be made about the learner's ability. The advantage of the Mini CEX is that it is used in a real-life setting and that the assessor can give rapid feedback to the learner to help them develop. As you might remember from Chapter 3, this does not often happen in the clinical environment and so has to be a good thing. On the downside, the original Mini CEX form is probably a little too generic for detailed, focused feedback in junior learners, and there have been some issues with actually getting people to fill them out.

Oral exams

Oral exams are part of the history and tradition of medical education and one way or another you might find yourself receiving a viva voce exam at the hands of two or three examiners. Institutions now tend to reserve these assessments for students at the borderline or students who might be worthy of a prize, although many have scrapped them entirely. If you take an intercalated BSc, you are still likely to have a viva on your thesis.

Traditionally, this form of exam has been received with terror from the candidates. The format is rather elegant: the examiners ask the student questions about a topic, with each question more difficult than the last, until they ascertain the upper limit of the candidate's knowledge on that topic, they then move to another topic and work up the ladder again. Within a relatively short time, they can build a picture of the candidate's depth of knowledge out of a range of core areas. Unfortunately, the frustrated candidate, regardless of whether they were good or bad, leaves the exam remembering only that they got the last question of every topic wrong and so tends to feel terrible.

Variations on a theme

So far in this chapter, we have tried to give an overview of the main assessment methods. Of course, there are many variations and the exams at your institution might be different. The OSCE, for example, looks a little different wherever you see it. Indeed sometimes people will take the OSCE concept and apply it to something else, such as an anatomy spotter exam, where students rotate around anatomy specimens answering questions or data interpretation exams where students rotate around radiographs, urine results and blood test results. Generally, people rename these exams anything that sounds like OSCE: OSPE, OSLER, OSTE – if you have a bored moment, try to make up some OSCE-like acronyms yourself and put them into PubMed. You are likely to find that someone else has come up with your acronym already! Similarly, Mini CEX, SAQs (short answer questions) and good old MCQs (multiple-choice questions) have all given birth to a multitude of variations. Our call from Chapter 10 remains – ensure that you understand the assessment programme at *your* institution, what it involves, what format it is in and what purpose it has.

Getting the best out of multiple-choice exams

MCQ exams, whatever the format, tend to strike fear into students' hearts. There are some simple rules to follow, though, which will make life much easier.

Manage your time effectively – use 'TimePosts'. Start the exam by looking through the question paper, check the number of questions and how much time you have for the exam. Work out how long you have to spend on each question (including any time you want left at the end for checking) and write next to every tenth question what time it should be when you reach that question. If you have already done most of the calculation before the exam, this should take less than a minute. These TimePosts will quickly flag up to you if you are running behind.

If you are filling in an automated marking grid, use these TimePosts as a reminder to check that you are still marking the question that you think you are marking. It is easy to skip a question and then all your answers refer to the question before or after the one you think you are answering. From personal experience, it is much better to discover that you have gone wrong early than when you get to the end of the exam!

There are no traps – if you are looking at a question not sure whether it means what it says or whether there is some secret second meaning in it, just go for what it says and move on. Having said that, **beware the double-negative question**: these are questions of dubious value that act as both a test of knowledge and a test of supreme logic at the same time. In Q14, double-negative answers *are* difficult to answer, so the statement in A is false and the question asks us 'which answer is false', so we highlight option A. For obvious reasons, most schools will now be avoiding double-negative questions, but one or two will sometimes slip through the net. Just go back to basics – look at the question, put a box around all the relevant words ('do not' and 'fall' in B) equates to 'stays the same or increases', this statement is true and so we do not select it).

Q14 One of the following statements is false:

A: Double negative questions are not difficult to answer.

B: Most liver enzymes do not fall in patients with hepatitis.

Sometimes there will be **badly written items** that might help give you some clues. Look for items that are much longer or shorter than their neighbours (in Q15, D is correct) and remember 'never' is always wrong, 'always' is never right', which is, of course, only a rule of thumb (very little in medicine is definite), so in Q16, you do not need to know much about items A, B, C and E to guess that they are false, leaving only item D as the correct one.

Q15 One of the following statements is correct
  The gene for cystic fibrosis is usually found:

A: On chromosome 1

B: On the X chromosome

C: On chromosome 5

D: On chromosome 7 and is responsible for coding for a regulation protein
   controlling ion and fluid flux across cell membranes

E: On chromosome 8

Q16 With respect to chest pain

A: Cardiac pain never radiates to the right arm

B: Cardiac pain is always described as crushing

C: Oesophageal pain is always burning in nature

D: Indigestion can sometimes resemble cardiac pain

E: Costochondritis never presents as pleuritic chest pain

Similarly, when answering **EMQs**, often there are not 11 or so good options, so the examiners might need to put in some clearly spurious ones. In Q10 and Q11 mentioned earlier, item K 'blood test' is clearly pointless, and indeed, some of the items clearly relate to very different sorts of questions. Clearly, questions about written exams could not possibly relate to a viva voce for example, which narrows your choices.

When answering EMQ questions, there is a process to go through (Figure 11.1). First read the stem – what is the question about? (For questions 10 and 11 you now know it is about forms of assessment.) Next read the question and see if an answer pops into your head. For question 10, you probably knew that the answer was true–false MCQ. Now look through the options, if it is there, write it down (option A). For question 11, you probably did not know the answer initially, so in this case you look through the options and see if the right answer is obvious. If you are still stuck, go through mentally or physically crossing off the answers that are clearly

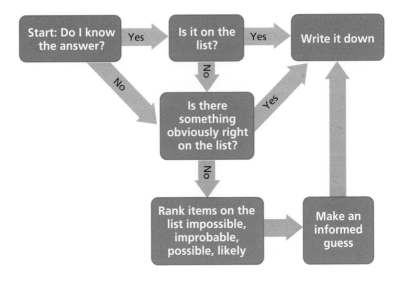

Figure 11.1 Process for answering extended matching questions.

wrong and see what you have left (bear in mind that you will need to look at them again, so do not deface the question paper too badly).

The most common mistake that students make with any form of multiple-choice exam is with their **preparation for the exam**. You will find a multitude of MCQs in books in the library and even more badly photocopied, barely legible lists of questions that someone you know has a friend who got them from someone who swore that they were real exam questions from some long-distant year. The mistake that people make is trying to memorise every question they come across. Your memory will not be able to hold all these questions and given a whiff of adrenaline in the exam, you will find that you can remember seeing the question before, or at least a question like it, but the answer, hmm, that is another question. This will lead to confusion and frustration. Even if you do have everything memorised, the chances are that the questions will not be identical to the ones you learned (examiners do not use books of exam questions to set the exams and they tend to rewrite, write new and edit existing questions in the bank of questions that your institution uses).

Past papers and external questions are really useful if you use them in the right way – namely for two functions. First, use them for timed mock exams to help you get used to the format and timing of the exam. Second, use them as a diagnostic tool. Look through your answers and when you get a question wrong, jot down the area that it relates to. If you get a couple of questions on similar topics wrong, that highlights a need for you to go back to your notes and revisit those topics. Remember, do not try and memorise answers to questions, go back and try and understand the topic.

Getting the best out of SJT exams

Revision and preparation

The same general advice applies as to all multiple-choice style questions, these have already been covered in pages 182–185. Mark 'Time Posts' (p. 168) on the question paper or on some rough paper to make sure that you pace yourself during the exam. Use these time posts or perhaps every tenth question to check that you are still scoring the mark sheet on the right question. Use a mental highlighter to pick out keywords in the question. Do not spend a disproportionate amount of time dwelling on difficult questions, as you will then run out of time and will not have answered many of the easier questions. In addition, of course, practise sometimes under exam conditions – you can even download a machine markable answer sheet to score your answers on. One other general principle that is particularly relevant: do not get too stressed about the exact ranking of individual items. Try and get it right, yes, but do not panic if you cannot decide whether items A and B should be ranked third and fourth or fourth and third – apply the following rules of thumb, but remember that thanks to the marking scheme if you get the question 100% right, you get 20 marks, but if you just transpose two items, you get a respectable 18 marks, if you get really stressed and panic, you will lose a lot more marks than that.

The SJT assesses that you know what you **should** do in various situations. This is how you are instructed to answer the questions – not on what you would do, but on what you think you **should** do. With this in mind, you clearly need some knowledge to answer the questions. For example, if you know that 'FY1 doctors should **never** discharge patients without close supervision' then you are likely to find it a lot easier to rank some of the items. You therefore should do some learning in preparation for the SJT, just as you would any other exam, but in this case you are not learning the management of diabetes, but instead learning **the roles and responsibilities of an FY1**. Sources that you might like to investigate are the GMC's Good Medical Practice (2013), the foundation programme curriculum and Appendix 1 of the SJT monograph (Patterson *et al.*, 2013). Remember to be curious on the wards, look up local and national policies on things like sick leave, dealing with bullying and so on, and remember that the choices that you see in practice do not necessarily reflect what an FY1 **should** do in those circumstances. You will also find the feedback from the sample online exam useful.

I thought I would do OK on the SJT, but after I did the online exam I realised that some of my expectations of the job were not right, and that I was answering a lot what I would do, rather than what I should do.

Tyler, final-year medical student.

I got feedback from the mock exam that 'it should not be necessary for anyone to work longer than their required hours because of what is essentially an organisational problem, not a medical emergency' – *this came as a bit of a shock to me, as my top answer for many of the questions was to stay late and sort problems out myself. This has made me realise that I'd made some assumptions about the examiners' expectations that were completely wrong.*

Jason, final-year medical student.

'**Read the question**' is a recurring theme in these chapters on assessment and it is particularly relevant for SJTs. Firstly, you need to ensure that you are clear on **what you are being asked to do**. For example, in ranking questions you may be asked a variety of different ways to rank (Table 11.1). As you can imagine, depending on this instruction, the same items could be ranked very differently. Secondly, when you read the scenario and items, be careful to stick with what they say. For those of us with a good imagination, the tendency is to embellish the story, reading 'between the lines' without even realising it – perhaps your colleague is late for work for this reason or that reason – this addition to the scenario ends up with you answering the question wrong. You must **respond only using the information given to you**. You will need to get into the habit of checking and double checking that you are answering the question as written rather than the question as you interpret them. Finally, when reading the question, **identify the key problem(s)/issue(s)** and consider the implication of each action, ensuring

Table 11.1 Be clear on what is being asked of you.

- Rank, in order, the appropriateness of the following actions in response to this situation: (1 = Most appropriate; 5 = Least appropriate)
- Rank, in order, the extent to which you agree with the following statements in this situation: (1 = Most agree with; 5 = Least agree with)
- Rank, in order, the importance of the following considerations in the management of this situation: (1 = Most important; 5 = Least important)
- Rank in the order that you should carry out the following steps in this situation: (1 = First; 5 = Last)

that they **address the problem**. For example, in one of the published sample questions, a stressed colleague might not be able to work this weekend. The priority is ensuring that there is *cover for this weekend*; so, in this scenario, suggest counselling is ranked quite low down the list of options, whereas in a different scenario it could come higher.

Table 11.2 lists some general rules of thumb for approaching SJT, you can probably add more to the list yourself.

Table 11.2 General rules of thumb for SJT.

- Something bad has happened – are you sure?
  - If you are certain that there is a risk to patient safety, you must act (patient safety always comes first)
  - If you are uncertain, you should investigate first (note the difference between hearsay –'someone tells you that your colleague has been drinking on duty' and fact 'you see your colleague drinking beer on duty')
  - Is there a sudden/acute risk? – if so then you need to take some form of action, if not, then you have time to investigate/consult
  - Address the immediate issue first, organisational change is relevant but usually comes later
  - Remember that you are only an FY1 and usually you would be expected to escalate concerns up the 'chain of command' rather than whistle-blowing straight to the top
- Things that are usually 'wrong'
  - Lying is always wrong, usually it is the 'most wrong' option
  - Anything that can be construed as gossip is usually wrong, and this might not be obvious, such as consulting colleagues on other teams about one of your team who is having difficulty. Sometimes this might be appropriate, but often not
  - Anything that might be seen to bring the profession into disrepute (see also Chapter 13 on professionalism)
- Things that are usually 'right'
  - Patient safety should 'always' come top of the list (there is no such thing as always in medicine, but this gets close)
  - Upholding trust in the profession is seen as important
  - An apology costs nothing – always apologise (but without blaming others and without adding a 'but')
  - Stand up for your team but do so diplomatically
  - In contrast to the aforementioned item, asking your peers for advice may well be appropriate, so long as it is not construed as gossip/destructive/vindictive
- For 'choose the three best answers' questions
  - Sometimes it helps to look for the 'least wrong' answers rather than the 'most right'
  - If you cannot decide on the third one to include between a couple of options, it often helps to choose the least controversial option

Chapter 11

Summary

SJTs are a relatively new form of assessment in medical education and can cause a lot of stress. Just as with any other form of assessment, they require core knowledge, an ability to apply this knowledge and a bit of exam technique. Not reading the question properly and reading between the lines of the scenario or options are both common causes of error. The foundation-year SJT questions go through a rigorous design and piloting process and are generally of high quality. The examples given here, and in many of the SJT 'revision' books, tend to be of more variable quality so use them with a critical eye and if you seriously disagree with a model answer, check with colleagues and faculty in your medical school, you might be right!

Acknowledgements

Many of the rules of thumb were generated within workshops done with final-year medical students at Kings College London in 2012 and 2013 as we worked through challenging example SJT questions. These students formed some fantastic study groups and we would very much recommend that you do the same.

Getting the best out of short answer questions

Our discussion of Q3 and Q6 in Chapter 10 highlights most of the key points about answering SAQs – read the questions carefully, box or highlight the key points and answer providing as much structure as possible to highlight the key points in your answer. You might consider 'counting out the answers': it is likely that if there are three marks for 'Describing the key findings likely on examination of a patient suffering from an myocardial infarction' (Q13 mentioned earlier), then the examiner is looking for three main points; unless, that is, the mark scheme gives half a mark for each main point, expecting six main points. Despite this difficulty, looking at the marks should help you structure your answer. If there is only one mark for a definition, then you might write a little less than if there were five marks for it.

We have already discussed the critical importance of strict timing and that you should answer every question that you are supposed to answer. We have also commented on planning. It is worth spending a minute or two planning out your answer: most schools would encourage you to include your rough plan in your answer, putting a single line through it to show that it is rough. If you run out of time, it might still earn you one or two marks.

If you read Chapter 2 (note taking) carefully, you will have a good idea of how to prepare for this form of exam. You can build writing your own questions into your day-to-day note taking and practise answering them as a way of reviewing your study. You will, of course, want to have full timed practice exams, but you should be very well prepared. Perhaps you will use a blend of your own questions and external ones. Perhaps you could share your questions with other students and build up a study group.

It is quite easy to test factual recall, and even understanding, with SAQ papers. It is much harder to write an SAQ that tests the more advanced skills that we discussed in Chapter 2, such as application, analysis and synthesis. It is possible for very skilled question writers to try and test these higher skills but, more often than not, these will be kept for other formats such as debates, vivas and, of course, the essay.

Getting the best out of the OSCE

It is likely that whatever your background, you will have had a fair amount of experience of a range of tests, but the OSCE is likely to be a new and rather daunting format. For this reason, we have added a rather generous section on OSCE performance.

The aim of the OSCE is simple. Imagine a geologist drilling down to take multiple core samples of the underlying soil and rock. At some point, he or she can say that enough samples have been taken to be able to build up a likely picture of what is underneath. If most/enough samples show clay, the under-lying soil is likely to be clay. In the OSCE, the concept is that an individual will demonstrate, through multiple samples, that they are competent across the breadth of necessary skills, so that the exam can infer that they are prob-ably competent across all skills. The aim of the exam, therefore, is to assess clinical competence – whether you will be any good at the job.

Students who strive to develop as good doctors, to learn the knowledge and skills required for the job and to become good at patient care, should pass the OSCE easily (with one or two caveats discussed in the following section). Unfortunately, some students see the OSCE as some kind of higher education hurdle unrelated to patients or being a doctor, and focus their learning not on becoming a good doctor, but on passing the exam. They work out elaborate schemes to 'perform well', but often will do badly.

Q17 You are a senior medical student in A&E. The registrar has asked you to take a venous blood sample to assess for anaemia. Please demonstrate how you would take blood, treating this rubber arm as if it were your patient.

Good students will have sought out many opportunities on the wards to take blood (with appropriate consent, of course, see Chapter 3), from time to time asking doctors, nurses or peers to watch them and check that they are doing it right. They will have become familiar with the different equipment available, including which bottles are used for which tests, they will have learnt rapport with patients when taking their blood and it is likely that they once forgot to write the patient's details on the sample and had to do them again with many apologies to the poor patient, and so they will never, ever do this again

In the exam, even on a rubber arm, these students will perform this skill fluently and professionally. It will be very obvious that they have done it many times before

This student passes the exam, but more importantly, you would be happy for them to take blood from your favourite aunt

The **exam-focused students**, knowing that the rubber arms used in the exam are not the same as real arms, will have practised mostly in the skills laboratory. They will have memorised a list of steps, perhaps from an OSCE book and practised reciting the steps with robotic reliability

Their training and practice, being focused only on the exam, will mean that in real life they are unlikely to be very good

In the exam, these students will be wooden in their performance, and may miss out steps that would be crucial in real life, but are less obvious in simulation (such as not remembering to write the patient's details on the bottle, or not knowing which bottle is used for which test)

This student probably fails the skill, or might scrape through, but most importantly, you would not let them anywhere near your favourite aunt with a needle

Looking at the two examples in Q17, it should be clear that those who strive just to pass the exam, to be OSCE competents, tend to perform worse in the exam than those who strive to become clinically (with patients) competent and who pass the exam as a 'side-effect'.

This is a crucial point and cannot be stressed enough. Ninety-five per cent of your learning of clinical and communication skills should be focused on becoming a great doctor, and perhaps 5% should be on exam technique. With a few tips on exam technique and a little bit of practice, you will then fly through the exam.

OSCE technique

Having said all this, there *are* times that students who do fairly well on the wards fall down in the OSCEs and this section aims to highlight common pitfalls and give some tips in dealing with them.

Suspension of disbelief

It is likely that you have watched a film that so engaged you that you felt part of it, that you were unaware of it as 'a film', but rather that it felt 'real'. At other times, you have watched a film and all you could see were shoddy actors on a screen. In your mind, you may have been critiquing the script, the direction, the sound track; it was far from 'real'.

There have probably been times that you have tried to move from one of these extremes to another – you noticed that you felt unengaged in the film and you took some steps to be drawn into it, or perhaps the film was so disturbing (perhaps a horror film that was too scary, or even an erotic moment in a film you watched with your parents) that you distanced yourself from what you were watching. Spend a minute and list down things that you have done to help you become drawn into the film and things that you have done to distance yourself (two columns). Go on, do it now, you probably need a break from reading anyway.

The OSCE is rather similar. Students who see it as an exam, something synthetic, a game perhaps, tend to have trouble engaging with it. Students who can imagine that each scenario is real, or at least who can 'suspend their disbelief' and approach each station as real, that the actor in front of them is a real patient, tend to do much better.

Q18 *You are a medical student in general practice. The GP has asked you to take a history from the next patient, Mr Leo Hill, who has been troubled recently with some chest pain. Please take a focused history in order to make a diagnosis. You have 5 minutes.*

Student A enters the station, shows her name badge to the examiner and sits down ensuring that the examiner is out of her line of sight. She introduces herself to the patient and imagines that he is, indeed, a patient in general practice. She asks him about his pain and as he is talking wonders what might be causing it. She naturally asks a blend of open (could you tell me a little more about the pain?) and closed (does the pain ever move down your arm?)

questions and summarises as she goes along to make sure she understands. She is curious about his thoughts about the cause and she discovers that he is very frightened that it might be from his heart. She can understand why that must be distressing, especially as his brother died recently from a heart attack. All in all, she takes a thorough history from the patient in front of her. She gets a real feel for how his symptoms are affecting him and thinks that she has excluded a cardiac cause and suspects that his symptoms might be due to acid reflux into the oesophagus or possibly a stomach ulcer.

When the bell goes and it is time to move on, the student is disoriented for a second. She had forgotten that she was in an exam. She gets her thoughts together, thanks the patient and moves on.

Student B enters the station and shows his name badge to the examiner. He notices the examiner holds the mark scheme and he wonders what is written on it. He knows that the first mark is likely to be for introducing himself so he turns to the actor and introduces himself in the way that he has practised for the OSCE. He watches the examiner from the corner of his eye to see if he ticks anything off on the mark scheme and, sure enough, it looks like he got a mark for the introduction – things have started well. He has found out a lot about past questions in this exam and wonders if this is the station from 2007 about cardiac pain or one from 2006 about acid reflux.

Knowing that the mark scheme will almost certainly reward using some open questions he asks 'Can you tell me about the pain?' and notices the examiner moving his pencil on the mark sheet – another point. The actor says 'Yes, it is quite frightening really. It tends to hurt just here', and points up and down the middle of the chest with the flat of his hand. The student knows than an actor would have been trained to use a fist if the pain was angina or a heart attack and feels pretty good about himself that he has identified that this is the acid reflux station from 2006, he smiles at the actor and says 'good'.

Somewhere else in the exam hall, he hears one of his colleagues saying in a loud voice 'I'd just like to examine your abdomen', and makes a mental note that there will be an abdominal examination station later in the circuit. His smile turns to a grin. He knows he has prepared for abdominal examination.

He asks the actor some more questions to show the examiner that he knows the diagnosis: 'Is it worse when you lie flat?' and 'Do you take milk and antacids and cimetidine to make it better?' The actor looks a little distressed but nods and the student smiles, seeing the perfect opportunity to gain a mark for empathy and says 'Yes, I know exactly how distressing this must feel for you.'

The student finishes early and sits back, trying to hear what the next station will be about. He hears the word 'warfarin' and smiles.

The **examiner** watched the two performances with interest. Her mark scheme rewarded students for taking a patient-centred history, for exploring the symptoms, for exploring all possible causes for chest pain and for being empathic and reassuring the patient appropriately. The first student did a very nice job and although she seemed to be less certain of a final diagnosis, she had explored all the right areas to exclude more serious causes of chest pain. She seemed to really care about how the patient felt. She got good marks and particularly gained marks for being fluent, professional and having a patient-centred approach. The second student did not score so well; indeed, his behaviour was rather odd. He did not ask the usual questions to exclude possible cardiac causes and seemed to jump straight to one diagnosis, asking nowhere near enough questions to confirm it safely. He smiled in the oddest places. He gained no marks for exploring the nature of the pain and no marks for exploring other possible causes. The examiner felt strongly that this candidate should not pass.

The actor was asked to mark each candidate for empathy. Although candidate A did not make any 'empathic statements', it was quite clear to him that she could really understand the patient's perspective and he scored her highly. He found candidate B rather bizarre: he smiled in odd moments and although he made an empathic statement, it was clear that there was no empathy behind it at all. He gave him zero marks.

You might think that this example (Q18) is unrealistic. Unfortunately, you would be wrong, OSCEs are too full of candidates 'playing the OSCE game' and losing out because of it. Look at your list from the exercise earlier. You probably identified some factors around focus and attention: you probably look away from the screen and focus on something typical of real life in order to escape the scenario, you might deliberately over-rationalise what you see (how ridiculous, that's not what someone would say in real life) and you might think of other things outside the film to bring you back to reality (what could you have for dinner?). To draw yourself in you might try and forget where you are, by ignoring distractions, positioning yourself perhaps to minimise distractions in your line of sight; you might also try and form an emotional connection with what you are watching – try and get into the lead actor's shoes, see how things are affecting him or her. You can use exactly the same skills in the OSCE – ignore distractions, focus on the patient and try and ignore the examiner. If you can position them out of your line of sight, all the better.

Chapter 11

You might want to practise gaining this focus. Perhaps you can role play some stations with your friends. When you get better at throwing yourself into the role required of you, perhaps you can try in environments where there are more distractions, such as the hospital canteen or even public transport. If you miss your stop on the train or bus because you were so engaged with finding out what was wrong with your 'patient', then you will know you are doing well. Consider things that might bring you out of focus, such as the examiner interrupting with a question, and practise how you can learn to manage these distractions and get back into the role quickly.

Read the question

OK, this should, by now, go without saying, but read the question. If you are told to take a history from the patient, do not start examining them and vice versa. If you are told to explain the mechanism of action, the potential benefits and the potential side effects of three drugs, you could see this is nine discrete tasks – do not leave any out. In most OSCEs, you will be given some time to read the task for each station before you enter the station and there is usually a copy of the task inside the station in case you forget. Examiners are trained not to prompt you, although most examiners will stop you if you start examining a patient's thyroid when you are only expected to talk to the patient and in these circumstances will usually ask you to read the question again.

Managing time

Some students are very good in clinical practice, but when it comes to the OSCE suddenly struggle because they keep running out of time. They might never have taken a 5-minute focused history in real life, or never just examined the nervous system of the legs in 5 minutes, and so they get stuck.

> 'Hello, my name is Peter Muthos; I'm a third-year medical student. I am just preparing for an exam and wondered if you would mind me practising by testing the nerves of your face. This would involve me just looking at your face, testing how strong the muscles around your head and neck are and seeing how sensitive to touch your skin is. I'd quite like to do this with my friend timing me for the exam. This is only for my learning, so no problem at all if you say no.'

Although 95% of your time practising should be spent on becoming clinically competent make sure that you spend some time practising timed scenarios. You can still do this with patients and if you get a peer to time you and give you feedback, you will learn a lot. You will feel a little rushed first off, but if you get fluent at taking a rapid, effective, focused, patient-centred history and conduct appropriate focused, diagnostic examinations, you will become a very popular junior doctor, especially in outpatient clinics, A&E and general practice.

Knowing triggers that distract you

We worked with a student who had been bullied by a teacher at secondary school. The teacher was a middle-aged woman with a disapproving look who taught gymnastics. She gave such withering, destructive feedback that our student, who wanted so much to do well in gymnastics, was usually brought to tears and eventually gave up. Years later in her first OSCE, she only had to see that a station had a middle-aged woman examining and she would freeze, heart pounding. She failed all stations where middle-aged women seemed to be judging her. She had some professional counselling and decided to face her fears. On the wards, she would tell female consultants that examiners who looked disapproving tended to put her off in the exam and asked if they might watch her examining a patient under exam conditions (she did not mention the middle-aged bit, in order to keep the consultants on her side). She became desensitised (although the first couple of times that she practised it was diffi-cult) and went on to do very well indeed in subsequent exams.

This example might seem extreme, but we all have triggers that can throw us in exams. Perhaps it is being interrupted in mid-flow, or the examiner ask-ing you to skip your usual starting steps of an examination and move straight on to the later steps, or perhaps it is the examiner yawning or looking uninter-ested. Whatever does it for you, learn what it is (see Chapter 7 on reflection) and actively engage in strategies to minimise its effect when you practise (remember if you are practising with patients, to include them in the deal – if your friend is going to interrupt you mid-flow with an unconnected question, you might want to let the patient know that you are practising how to manage distractions, otherwise they will think something very odd is going on).

Dealing with 'brain freeze'

Every student's dread in an OSCE is that they will completely dry up: after years of preparation, after seeing hundreds or even thousands of patients, they walk into a station, or get halfway through a station, and their brain turns to a mush that is barely able to keep them breathing, let alone hold anything that resembles a thought. Mouth open, heart pounding, panic wells up from the guts, but still no thoughts arrive.

As we discussed earlier, this is pure and simple stage fright; it is common and, in fact, normal. If you recognise what it is, accept it as normal and learn to actively manage it, you will be fine. If you pretend it will never happen to you, when it does happen, you will be in trouble.

Talk to other people who have done OSCEs at medical school and ask them for tips on managing brain freeze. You could even collate your findings and offer them to others. There are some common strategies that we describe here, but we are sure that you can find out many more.

- **Summarise**: it will show that you know what is going on and usually the next thing to do becomes obvious; for example, 'If I could just summarise, you got this chest pain last night, it came on after exercise, went down your left arm and it was crushing in nature, is that right? Can I go on and ask, did anything make it better?'
- **Invite questions**: this will buy you some time, will get you saying something sensible rather than just saying 'ummmmm' and drooling and might open up some more avenues; for example, 'I realise that I have been asking you a lot of questions, I wonder if you have any questions or concerns for me?'
- **Ask open questions**: for example, a simulated patient (actor) has just told you that they have a certain disease and you cannot quite place that disease for the moment – your mind has gone blank. Hopefully, their answer will trigger you to remember. 'Gosh, that's interesting, how does the myasthenia gravis tend to affect you?'
- **Move to 'safer' ground**: sometimes you might feel uncomfortable or lost on one part of the history, such as the history of the main problem (history of presenting problem). You might decide to move on to an area that you feel more comfortable in order to gain confidence before going back. 'Could I just move on and ask you something about your family history? Are both your parents well?' This approach can lead to a disjointed consultation, but is better than staring at the patient in silence waiting for the right bit of information to pop into your head.

You will need to practise these strategies both with real patients and with friends in simulation so that in an exam, if you get brain freeze, you can quickly grab a semi-automatic rescue strategy without having to expend much thought.

Leaving each station behind

You will do badly on some of your OSCE stations. This is a simple fact and as the final OSCE marks tend to be averaged across all the stations, you can afford to do badly in a few stations. Some students do badly in a station and then cannot think of anything except that station; they keep thinking back about other things that they could have said or done and as a result they under-perform on the next station and then the next station.

The simple truth is that students rarely know how they did on a station. Basic skills, such as examining a patient's respiratory system, usually have a high pass mark. Students leave these stations thinking they did well (they did most of it right), but actually did not do as well as would be expected (they were expected to do all of it right). In contrast, students often leave really challenging stations thinking they have done badly, but actually they were not expected to do well, so the pass mark for that station might be very low. You might well fail stations that you think you did well in and pass stations that you think you did badly in.

Some students find it quite challenging to move from thinking about one skill straight into thinking about another with very little time in between. Practise a few 5-minute skills in a row and get used to going from one skill to a completely different skill – it can be disorienting the first couple of times.

Start a ritual that will help you leave each station behind you and allow you to focus on the next task in hand. Make it a ritual that is personal to you. Perhaps at each new station you smile and shake hands with the examiner or patient, perhaps you can see the ritual of introducing yourself as, in some way, purifying you from the last station. You might find some physical stress relief techniques to help, such as clenching your fist really tightly, feeling all the tension go into that fist, feel it getting tighter and tighter and then shaking it loose, feeling the tension dissipate (with practise you can do this subtly and in between stations, as it is probably best not to shake your fist at the examiner, nor the next patient!). Breathing exercises, brief visualisations, there are endless possibilities: find something that works for you and practise it until you can do it automatically when stressed.

Saying 'I don't know'

Every day, senior clinicians say 'I don't know' to patients. The thing that differentiates them from junior medical students is that they tend to say something along the line of 'I don't know, but let me find out some more information from you and then this is my plan for finding out and getting back to you'. What doctors do not do (should not do) is lie to patients, make things up in order to answer their questions. Imagine the following OSCE station:

Q19 *You are a senior medical student on a surgery attachment. Your team is referring the next patient for an upper gastrointestinal endoscopy. Please explain the procedure to the patient.*

Student C: 'Hello there, my name is . . . I understand that you have been referred for an endoscopy, and I have been asked to come and explain it to you. I must say that I am not an expert on the subject but I thought that I could

> find out what you understand already, and what your main questions are, then I could explain as best I can and if there are any outstanding questions I will either find out myself and come back to you, or I will ask one of my seniors to come and talk to you. Would that be all right?'
>
> **Student D** (makes up incorrect facts): 'Ah well, yes, hmm, an endoscopy – well, we will pass a big telescope down your throat, erhm, but don't worry, you will be put to sleep first, hmmm, and we will keep you in overnight to make sure you are afterward [pause] ah yes, risk, hmm, well, no risk at all, very safe, unless, hmm, well, no, it is completely safe.'

For some reason, some (sometimes many) students think that it is OK to lie in an OSCE. True enough, saying 'I don't know' and sitting silent for the next 4 minutes and 50 seconds does not do you any favours, but admitting uncertainty finding out the patient's perspective and prior knowledge and proposing a plan for getting the information that you do not know back to the patient really will.

Pulling it together

The last section on OSCEs has been lengthy, but only really has two messages. The first is to throw yourself into the role as if each station is a real-life scenario – read the student brief for the station and imagine that it is true. Try and avoid the temptation to second guess the examiner. The second is to consider possible challenges for you in the exam (running out of time, freezing etc.) and ensure that, as well as practising in order to be a competent doctor, you also spend a little time practising OSCE technique with your peers.

Getting the best out of workplace-based assessments (WPBA)

> *"The medical school makes me do four Mini-CEX on each placement, it's just a tick box exercise. I end up always doing them in the last week – I can usually find someone to just sign me off. I really don't see the point"*
>
> Selina, final-year medical student.

There is a simple choice you must make about how you want to use workplace-based assessments (WPBA) (Mini-CEX, DOPs etc.): **either** you can see them as a hurdle/tick box exercise that you need to get past (with the minimum of effort) to progress, **or** you can see them as a fantastic opportunity for learning and to get feedback.

When done right, WPBA ensure that students are observed performing skills and given focused feedback by a clinician (and we know that both of these events are often very rare in a medical student's training). They allow students to monitor and plan their progress, and help them reflect not only on areas where they need to improve, but also gain awareness of the things that they do really well and so should not change. Unfortunately, WPBA are often not done right and so have little benefit.

The London Deanery for postgraduate training (now renamed 'SharedServices' but still easier to find by putting 'London Deanery' into a search engine) propose a useful acronym to encourage the effective use of WPBA – Trainees should be SAFER. They should:

- Spread assessments through the attachment – that way you get feedback early, gaps are identified early and you can see how you develop during the attachment. You do not need to pass every assessment on the first attempt and you are certainly not expected to demonstrate competence as a junior medical student. **Do not** leave the assessments all until the last minute and then panic to get them completed.

- As many assessors as possible – they will all give you slightly different types and different focus of their feedback to you, some will be a bit too critical and others will not be critical enough – a good spread will give a good balance. Some will focus more on your communications skills, others on your clinical skills and so on. Do not forget that your assessors usually do not always need to be doctors. For many skills, nurses or other health-care professionals may be just as good, or often better, to observe, give you feedback and complete the relevant assessment form.

- Feedback as well as scores – many of the forms have numerical scores, often ranging from 1 to 9 with a space for written feedback. Students and trainees get very worked up about the exact score, with one consultant maybe giving mostly sevens and another giving mostly eights. Our view is that the numbers are useful, but ONLY as a trigger for feedback – if you got a 7 for communication, why was it not a 6 (what did you do well)? And why was it not an 8 (what could you have done better)? It is, therefore, the feedback and not the score that is the most useful aspect of WPBA. Indeed, the foundation years WPBA are all shifting to focus completely on feedback rather than scores.

- Evidence – ask for specific examples of what you did, keep a record and review how you develop, make sure that the feedback is written down or else you *will* forget it.

Chapter 11

- Reflect on what you did, how you are developing and what you need to do next.

> *"I often feel a bit shy asking a busy doctor to watch my clinical skills. The fact that I have to have five Mini-CEX completed on each firm is a good excuse for asking someone to watch me and give me feedback. All the junior doctors have to do them too, so it is seen as just part of the job"*
>
> Mirko, fourth-year medical student.

Although WPBA, when done correctly, can be a fantastic opportunity for learning, when done badly they can have unpredicted side effects. Imagine you are shadowing a junior doctor. He offers to watch you take blood and complete a DOPS (direct observation of practical skill) assessment for you. He does so and comments what an excellent medical student you are. You ask him if he would mind filling out some of your Mini-CEX forms as well, because although he has not observed you, he knows you are OK and you have to do a whole bunch of them before the end of your attachment next week. At first glance, this may seem reasonable. Thinking a little more deeply, in this scenario, you are asking a professional to lie on your behalf. Not only to lie, but also to state that they have observed you and believe that you are safe and appropriate with patients, assessing your ability to practice as a professional, when they have not. This would not only bring into question their probity in general (signing something that is not true), but also their commitment to ensuring juniors and colleagues are fit to practice and hence the entire philosophy of revalidation. This would be a serious breach of their professionalism (and indeed doctors have been suspended by the GMC for doing this), and in asking them to do so would be a serious breach of your professionalism. We have added a whole chapter on professionalism, to help you navigate through a terrain that can initially seem rather unclear (Chapter 13)

The viva

As we mentioned earlier, vivas are getting less common these days. Knowing the structure and format helps (the fact that they will always ask up to your level of 'not knowing', see the earlier section, means that you can remain confident even though you get things wrong).

Probably the most important skill in answering a viva is to structure your answer well.

Q20 *Tell me about ruptured ectopic pregnancy.*

Student P: 'Hmm, well, erhm, it's where a pregnancy forms in the fallopian tube, erhm, usually around 6 weeks of pregnancy, erhm, it can be quite dangerous...'

Student Q: 'Ruptured ectopic pregnancy is a gynaecological emergency, it is managed by making a rapid diagnosis through history, examination and special investigations carried out while concurrently resuscitating the patient, followed by emergency surgical treatment. The features on the history that would identify this diagnosis would be...'

In this example (Q20), student P has actually given more hard facts than student Q, but student Q has started with confidence (without actually saying much), has set the scene (making it clear that this is an emergency) and has laid out a plan for continuing to answer the question (he will talk about history, examination, special investigations, resuscitation and surgical treatment). Through giving this answer and signposting each time he moves on to a separate part of the answer, he will convince the examiner that he is a clear thinker who understands the information. Some examiners might even move him on after that introduction to another topic, believing that he has already demonstrated that he knows more than enough about this topic.

If vivas are likely in your curriculum, it would be a good idea to get plenty of practice, by recording yourself to practise fluency and structuring your answers, using your peers to practise answering unexpected questions and using any faculty who have experience in 'vivaring' to practise how you would handle it in real life. Developing these skills will be useful in later life for job interviews and so on.

Summary

Chapters 10 and 11 have tried to highlight some of the common pitfalls found in assessment at medical school and how to avoid them. Good exam technique in no way replaces appropriate learning, but rather goes hand-in-hand with it. Hopefully, the tone of this book in general and the section on OSCEs in particular has highlighted that the purpose of medical school is to prepare you to become an excellent doctor. Exams are part of that journey, but should not be seen as the destination.

Chapter 11

References and further reading

Your library will have books on exam technique, especially essay writing, and some great resources on referencing and plagiarism. We have found the following books useful.

Cottrell, S. (2006). *The Exam Skills Handbook: Achieving Peak Performance.* Basingstoke, Palgrave Macmillan.

Evans, M. (2004). *How to Pass Exams Every Time.* Oxford, How To Books.

Foundation Programme Curriculum – www.foundationprogramme.nhs.uk/Pages/home/training-and-assessment

GMC Good Medical Practice, 2013.

Lewis, R.S. (1993). *How to Write Essays.* London, National Extension College.

Patterson, F., Ashworth, V. & Good, D. (2013). *Appendix 1 of Situational Judgement Tests: A guide for applicants of the UK Foundation Programme.* Medical Schools Council & Work Psychology Group.

Questions and answers

Q: However hard I try, I cannot do well on multiple-choice questions. I often go back and change my answers when I read through them again. Is that the right thing to do?

A: MCQ papers can be challenging. Some students tend to answer more questions right the first time and then become indecisive and 'correct' them to become wrong answers when they look back at the end. Other students tend to improve their score by checking. Do some practice questions and note down which answers you change. Tot up your score before and after making changes and see what the difference is for you. Do this for a few mock exams and you should see a pattern emerging.

Q: I understand that I should not copy out someone else's text from their work and not attribute it to them, but it is OK to paraphrase, isn't it?

A: If you use someone's ideas, you must reference. Descartes said: 'I think, therefore I am.' Even if you paraphrase to 'I think, therefore I exist' it remains his idea, and not yours. Paraphrased plagiarism is harder to detect than 'cut and pasted' plagiarism, but is no less wrong.

Q: In a multiple-choice question paper, should I leave the questions I am not sure of blank to come back to or should I guess?

A: This depends on the sort of exam, the amount of time and your personal preference. In general, it is better to answer everything as you go along, leaving none blank. This makes it easier to time accurately and helps reduce the risk of you getting out of sync between the question sheet and the mark sheet. If you are allowed to rub out answers, then mark the question sheet to highlight the ones that you have guessed, so that you can go back.

Chapter 12 **Teaching, mentoring and coaching: helping others to learn and develop**

Education is the kindling of a flame, not the filling of a vessel

Often attributed to Socrates (c. 470 BC – 399 BC)

OVERVIEW

This chapter, new for the second edition, shifts focus away from your learning and development, onto the ways that you can help others learn and develop. These are core life-long skills for doctors and are increasingly formalised in undergraduate and postgraduate curricula. In the United Kingdom, this is formalised within GMC documentation, BMA guidance (see the following section) and the foundation school curriculum.

In this chapter, we cover some basics of teaching, linking how to help others learn with the chapters on how to learn yourself. We discuss lesson planning, how to evaluate the quality of your teaching and highlight some of the potential unwanted effects of teaching that you may deliver. In the second half of this chapter, we discuss mentoring and coaching, and how these concepts can be applied giving mentoring and/or coaching to others, receiving mentoring and/or coaching from others or making a reciprocal arrangement work.

… The word 'doctor' means physician, and is derived from the Latin *docere*, to teach. All doctors in the UK are required to teach future generations of doctors, yet, unlike the preparation provided for their roles as clinicians and despite their expertise in what they teach, there has

How to Succeed at Medical School: An Essential Guide to Learning, Second Edition. Dason Evans and Jo Brown.

traditionally been a deficiency in appropriate teacher education in the medical profession.

(British Medical Association Board of Medical Education, 2006)

Introduction

This is principally a book on how to learn, however, we felt in the second edition that it would be worth giving a brief introduction to teaching. The reasons for this are twofold: firstly, although medical students have always taught, coached and mentored their peers informally, increasingly medical schools are formalising these programmes. In some medical schools, students are even paid by the school to teach their peers or their juniors. The second reason to include something on teaching here is to highlight that there is a continuum between learning and teaching – teaching is, after all, simply helping others to learn.

There are three fundamental educational philosophies (Table 12.1), which form different camps. Generally, we have moved on from the behaviourist tradition, as seeing the learner as some kind of leaky bucket who needs to be filled up with facts faster than they can leak out, towards cognitive and constructivist approaches. We no longer think of teaching as passing on facts to the learner, but instead as a much more active process, where learning is constructed in the learner's mind. In reality, we commonly use principles from all three philosophies, although you could easily plan some teaching that used purely one approach or another, for the same topic. Perhaps you might give that a go and see which the learners prefer?

Unfortunately, definitions of teaching have not really kept up with the times; however, one that we like from www.OxfordDictionaries.com is

Cause (someone) to learn or understand something by example or experience.

This chapter is light on theory. There is a massive body of educational theory out there and teaching without attention to the theories behind how people learn is a little like surgery without attention to the knowledge around anatomy – often things will go wrong and you will not know why! If you find this chapter interesting, why not consider contacting your local department of medical education and asking if you can do a project in Med Ed, or even consider an intercalated bachelors or masters' degree? We have added a couple of straightforward texts under *Further Reading* that you might find an easy introduction.

Table 12.1 Three educational philosophies.

Behaviourist approaches

- The learner is seen as a passive recipient, with emphasis on the teacher. Learning is analogous to the development of a habit through repetition and practice. Learning is demonstrated by a change in performance. Reinforcement, positive and negative feedback are important
- Examples include much e-learning – where there is a pre-test, you are given information and then a post-test. Traditional lectures where the lecturer is the 'sage on the stage' who is unaware of the audience and the learners just sit and make notes. Learning a clinical skill by rote, through repetition with feedback (drill)

Cognitivist approaches

- Emphasis on promoting mental processes. Learning is an active process so the learner is central to the process. Much of Chapter 2 reflects cognitivist approaches to learning (learning for recall, contextual learning, linking new knowledge to old knowledge etc.)
- Examples include interactive workshops, well designed, interactive lectures, some forms of problem-based learning

Constructivist approaches

- These approaches see knowledge being created by how the individual (or group) creates meaning from his or her own experiences. This occurs through an interaction of activity, existing knowledge and context/culture. Group learning, discussion triggered by respectful discussion around difference of opinions, contextualised learning, 'authentic tasks anchored in meaningful contexts'
- Examples include teaching and learning of anything that does not have a concrete definition – how do students learn professionalism? Professional identity? Teaching includes principles of teaching in context, application of knowledge, facilitating true self-directed learning (i.e. objectives truly set by the learners, not by the teachers)

Adapted from Ertmer, P. A. and T. J. Newby (1993). 'Behaviorism, cognitivism, constructivism: Comparing critical features from an instructional design perspective.' *Performance Improvement Quarterly 6(4)*, 50–72.

An introduction on how to teach

The continuum of learning and teaching: 'teaching for learning'

This is not a book on how to teach (although we plan to write one, one day), but as peer teaching becomes increasingly formalised, we thought that it would be useful to include this brief introduction. The secret, that no one ever tells new teachers, is that there is a continuum from learning to teaching. This book is principally about how to learn, but that translates well into how to approach teaching as well; teaching is, after all, simply a process that encourages learning. See Table 12.2 for examples.

Chapter 12

Table 12.2 The continuum between learning and teaching.

	Learning	Teaching	Example
Motivation is core to learning	It is important to work out what motivates you and adapt how you learn to maximise motivation (e.g. Chapter 1 and positive spirals in Chapter 3)	It is important to work out what motivates the learner(s) and adapt how you teach to maximise their motivation	Teaching the anatomy of the anterior triangle of the neck, do you want to introduce the topic by saying 'look, this is a bit dry, but it is important and I will try and make it as easy to remember as possible' or 'OK, imagine you are in the Emergency Department and a patient comes in with a knife through the base of their neck. Before you remove it, you need to know exactly which structures might be involved – that's what we are going through in this session.'?
Deep learning is characterised by understanding and results in better long-term recall	Try to make learning active, focusing on understanding via examples, application and linking in with prior knowledge	Try to make learning active, focusing on developing understanding via examples, application and linking in with prior knowledge	Get the learners to brainstorm on what they know about a topic before teaching (activate prior knowledge), explicitly link your teaching to this prior knowledge, ask them to apply what they are learning to different scenarios in order to ensure that they understand. Do everything you can to create active engagement and discourage passive observation
Learning in context results in improved recall in that context	Try and apply what you are learning to real life problems/scenarios	Try and get them to apply what they are learning to real life problems, use patient scenarios, multiple different examples, consider making simulation as realistic as possible	Teaching cardiovascular examination on a volunteer – ensure that the volunteer is correctly positioned, make sure that everyone washes their hands just as they would with a patient and treat the volunteer just like a patient (even if they are a colleague) – especially with respect to maintaining patient dignity, communication skills and behaving professionally.

Chapter 12

Encouraging life-long learning	It is essential for medical students to develop a habit of life-long learning (Chapter 2). In this book, we encourage you to seek out problems, to work out yourself what you need to know and to what depth (using evidence and advice to inform your judgements), to work out the best way to learn (and build a toolkit of different active approaches to learning) and to feel ownership of what you learn; feeling good about yourself for what you have learned	Fostering these feelings in others requires you to move away from older concepts of teaching (the sage on the stage) to someone who may leave some niggling questions open to encourage students to read further, to encourage ongoing practice and to help the learners think about how they will ensure that they keep up to date in a changing landscape. Excellent teaching will help learners develop their study skills and an awareness of which ones are best to use when	Clinical skills are learnt by a combination of knowledge (the steps, the basic science behind the steps and two different types of clinical reasoning), practice (10 000 hours to develop expertise) and feedback, all influenced by the learner's frame of mind (Chapter 3). When teaching clinical skills, you might only have time to cover the steps, a little bit of practice and a bit of feedback. If the learners' leave the session thinking that they now know the skill, they will be really grateful and you will feel great about yourself, but it will not be true. They will not be competent for a long while yet and will not become expert without years of deliberate practice. You must ensure that they leave the session knowing that there is a lot more work to do and with a plan for how they will continue to learn and improve at the skill
Other examples	You could re-read this whole book, particularly Chapters 1–4, asking yourself 'How can I utilise these principles when I teach?'		

Chapter 12

Before teaching

Lack of planning is the commonest error in teaching. The plan does not need to take a long time to create, but it ensures that you have thought about the audience and you have considered the level and what you want them to learn. It will give you some structure and so make the session flow more logically.

A learning needs assessment (Figure 12.1) allows you to pitch at the right level, not losing them in complexity or boring them covering old ground. It allows you to link new learning to old learning and so maximise motivation, encoding information into memory and recall. Your learning needs assessment may be as simple as knowing your audience and their curriculum, or may be as interactive as starting your session with a quiz or clinical scenario.

The plan can be as complete as Gangé's (Table 12.3) or as simple as the plan shown in Figure 12.2: an Introduction, Body and Summary, with timings added and some details under each heading. A good plan allows you paradoxical flexibility, if you end up spending a little longer on one part than intended, this should be clear from your plan so that you can cut down elsewhere.

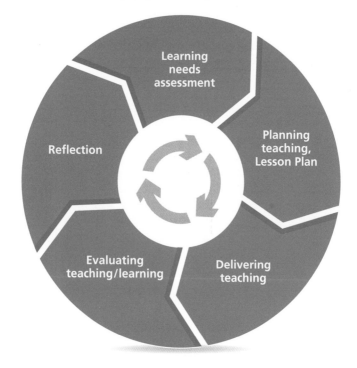

Figure 12.1 The teaching cycle.

Time	Structure	Teacher activity	Student activity	Resources and comments
	Introduction	**"OMMUCK"** O : give clear Objectives – setting expectations on content and level M : attend to student Motivation M : set the Mood U : Utility – how will this be useful? C : Content – what is going to be covered K : activate their prior Knowledge	May include brainstorming, answering questions, group-work etc.	
	Body	Fill this with the order that things will be covered. Remember that 1 : you are teaching for learning, so use active principles 2 : you can't cover everything, if you try they will be overloaded and not remember anything 3 : the order that you cover things in may be important to build up a story, as will the strategies in which you do so		Resources that you will use Perhaps also reminders of anecdotes that you can tell, or common misconceptions or myths that you need to dispel
	Close	A summary, covering no new content is often useful to review the intended objectives, utility and content, and then discuss the next steps with the learners		

Figure 12.2   A basic Lesson Plan. Adapted from WK Kellogg Foundation, Center for Learning Resources (1975). *TIPS: The Teaching Improvement Project System.* University of Kentucky, Kentucky, USA.

Chapter 12

Chapter 12

Table 12.3 Gagnés' instruction events.

Stage	Explanation	Examples
Setting the stage		
1. Motivate	• Gain the learner's attention and trigger their motivation. Internal motivation (wanting to learn for interest/curiosity or for patient care etc.) is much stronger than for exams and exam focus can handicap deep learning – so avoid discussion of OSCEs • Different people have different triggers for motivation	• Use patient scenarios or examples from your own experience ('I saw a patient who had been knifed in the base of the neck, I was really glad that I had learnt the regional anatomy' or 'back pain is so common that it is really essential to know how to examine the back and exclude red-flag signs of serious pathology') • Consider linking to basic science (learning about the different features of valvular heart disease can really help you learn cardiovascular physiology) • Try and keep comments motivating and avoid things like 'neuro exam is really difficult, I doubt you'll ever get it' or 'learn this now, no one will ever help you on the wards'
2. Explain target objectives/ level for session	• Students who aim too high or too low during the session will become frustrated and disappointed. It is unrealistic, for example, for a student to master a fluent neurological examination in their first ever session on neurology	• 'Today is about introducing you to the principles of the motor neurological examination – particularly observation, tone, power, reflexes and coordination. I'm not expecting anyone to be perfectly fluent at the end of the session – you'll have to carry on practising – but I hope that we can get the steps all clear and get you all able to do each part right'
3. Stimulating prior recall	• All learning is linked to prior knowledge, activating this prior knowledge will result in much deeper learning	• There are many different ways of activating prior knowledge • Brainstorm on the whiteboard what they know already • Ask questions based on basic science, clinical science or even general knowledge (Who here has had their blood pressure measured? OK, talk us through, what did they do first? ....) • **Avoid** questions that are easy to close down – Q: 'What do you know about BP?' A: 'Nothing' Q: 'OK, let me start from the beginning ...'

Core learning activities

4. Demonstrate key features
- A real-time run-through of the skill
- You might want to stick to the basics
- A real time run-through of a 5-minute motor examination of the upper limbs

5. Individualise
- Break it down according to the level of the learners
- Link steps backward to basic science and forward to clinical reasoning
- Add in more advanced practice if appropriate
- Demonstrate and talk through observation, ask the group to prompt you for the sort of things that might indicate pathology, show the two or three main approaches to assessing tone … etc.
- Identify key points such as isolating one muscle group (which muscle group, which nerve root?) when testing power

6. Elicit practice
- Hands-on practise is **essential** for learning a skill
- All members of the group should practise. Consider tactics for getting everyone to have a go
- Either whole task (practising whole motor exam)
- Or part task (show tone, practise tone, feedback on tone, then show them power, practise power, feedback on power …)
- Consider splitting the group into three's (patient, 'doctor' and observer) and getting them to rotate tasks.

7. Feedback
- Constructive feedback (aimed at helping improvement) is essential for learning
- Use the group to provide feedback to each other wherever possible, with you summarising and covering important issues that have been left out
- Providing feedback while the learner is doing is better for novices. As the learner becomes more fluent, save your feedback for the end
- Most people can only remember three points of feedback, so avoid the temptation to tell them everything
- Consider giving group members specific feedback tasks (e.g. one watches communication with the patient, one comments on technical aspects, another on fluency and one on infection control)
- There is some evidence that if you ask the learner their impressions first and then build feedback on their self-perception that their learning will be deeper

(continued overleaf)

Table 12.3 *(continued)*

Stage	Explanation	Examples
Rounding up		
8. Assess performance	• Ideally have one final run-through, or if no time, make a comment about where the group has reached today • Consider basing your feedback on the target objectives for the session • No new information	• 'Ok, so we were aiming to get everyone comfortable with assessing tone, power, reflexes and coordination. Most people are there with everything apart from reflexes, which seem to need a lot more practise, particularly triceps …'
9. Encourage ongoing practise and transfer	• 10 000 hours of practice are required to develop expertise. This teaching session is just a drop in the ocean in comparison • **The** most important teaching intervention you can do is to motivate them to continue to practise and get effective feedback from each other • Help them consider how they will put what they have learnt into practice when they hit the wards	• 'Fantastic, so a little more work is needed for reflexes and a lot more work is needed before you become slick – when are you going to practise this next? Is it worth arranging a time when the whole group will get together?' • 'Whenever I examine a patient I always add neuro exam into the full examination – it takes longer to begin with but I'm now much faster' • 'The elderly care wards are great places to practise neuro exams – lots of patients with signs and usually they are quite bored and pleased to see students'

Modified for peer tutoring of clinical skills. Adapted from O'Connor, H. M. (2002). 'Training undergraduate medical students in procedural skills.' *Emergency Medicine (Fremantle)*, *14(2)*, 131–135

When planning teaching, be aware that if you know a topic or skill really well, you may actually have some trouble teaching it – make sure you can deconstruct the topic into small bites so that novices can easily follow.

Teaching methods/delivering teaching

You have probably done quite a bit of teaching already. When you explain something that you understand to your peers who do not, then you are teaching. Explaining something to patients is a form of teaching. When you give directions to a stranger in the street, you are teaching. When you ask your nephew what he did at school today and then enthusiastically ask him how that could be applied in real life, you are teaching.

Teaching, therefore, does not require PowerPoint, or learners sitting in rows facing you and you have already experienced teaching, probably without knowing it. There are, however, some general principles, which are nicely summarised by Gagné's Instructional Events. In Table 12.3, we have included a summary of these, including an explanation and examples. This table was created originally by Dason Evans for the peer tutor programme at St Georges, where carefully selected, trained, monitored and paid senior students deliver clinical skills teaching to junior students, as part of the core curriculum. It has since been edited and modified for many different student and staff teaching, including JASME (the medical student and junior doctors group of the Association for the Study of Medical Education), and has been used around the world. Thanks are owed to too many to mention for their various tweaks and improvements. The original document is based on an easy-to-read and freely available article (O'Connor, 2002, see *Further Reading*), and Gagné's book originally published in 1965, which is a little less accessible. This summary specifically addresses clinical skills, but can easily be adapted to teaching knowledge. You will see that Gagné's approach closely follows what we know about learning.

After teaching

Evaluation

After teaching, you should ask yourself three questions:

- 'Was it any good? How do I know?' (i.e. did they learn effectively?)
- What are the things that I did that worked well?
- What should I change if I ran it again?

Evaluating the quality of teaching is actually not an easy thing to do; however, in Table 12.4, we have listed some suggestions for approaches that you

Table 12.4 A range of approaches to evaluating teaching.

Method	Examples
Self-reflection	Reflective learning diaries – see the following
Quantitative student evaluations	Likert Scales (I found the presentation clear SA/A/N/D/SD) Please rate the quality of this teaching on a scale of 0–10
Qualitative student evaluations	What were the three most useful things about this course? What were the three least useful?
Peer observation of teaching	A colleague comes and watches my teaching after a discussion about my rationale and concerns about the approach that I use. After the teaching, the colleague gives me useful feedback and advice
Attendance	I watch for trends in student attendance over the course, if they come I must be good
Testing students	Example 1: Before I teach I give a short MCQ and after I teach I give a similar one to see if the students have learnt anything Example 2: I ask students to demonstrate a neurological examination before and after my teaching on the topic
There are many other approaches	

might use. In best practice, you would triangulate several different approaches to come up with a judgement. If you decide to use learner questionnaires, which is one of the commonest forms of evaluation, then think about what you want to know from them and then either go searching on the Internet, where you will find thousands of different teaching evaluation questionnaires, or create your own. Keep these forms safe, they will go in your portfolio (Chapter 7) and provide good evidence of teaching.

Reflection and planning for next time

Consider writing some brief notes directly after the teaching session. What do you think went well, what were you less happy with? What objectives did you have at the start – do you think that you managed to address them all adequately?

If there were any significant or unexpected events, then describe what happened, list all the possible explanations that could have led to the event and all the possible solutions you could have applied (including prevention before and reaction after), now write down what you did and what you might try next time.

Motivation for teaching, curriculum considerations and unexpected outcomes

In Chapter 1, we asked you why you wanted to be a doctor and acknowledged that there were many different reasons, and different people have different motivations. Similarly, why would someone want to teach? Why would *you* want to teach? Some want to improve patient care: they teach using a lot of patient examples, refusing to talk about exams; others like to see students learning as a result of their interventions, they will ask students to solve problems, glow with pride when they can and get frustrated when they cannot solve them. Some are almost addicted to getting students to that light bulb or 'aha' moment when they suddenly understand something complex, they tend to ask lots of questions that challenge students to build links and think about things in different ways. There are some who teach to feed their egos, to have the eternal gratitude of their students – they tend to give students the impression that their teaching session is all that they need; they tend to teach for the exams, 'listen to me and you will do fine'. There are lots of different motivators and, in truth, all teachers probably have a combination of most of them. It is worthwhile considering, what is *your* main motivation for wanting to teach others?

Believe it or not, your medical school curriculum will have an underlying philosophy. It might be explicit and well thought out or it might be more implicit. If the curriculum has recently been renovated, then most sessions will follow it and if it is getting a bit tired, there will have been some drift. Medical School A has a philosophy that teaching is central to learning. They have experts in most fields and a curriculum that, in the early years, revolves around lectures and seminars, teaching basic science as a pure science, informed by internationally renowned researchers. The core curriculum is well defined and exams expect students to have excellent factual knowledge, as the school believes that a good grounding in the sciences will lead to the production of more academically informed doctors. The students get stressed in the second half of the year about the exams and a group of senior students start revision lectures. Some of these lectures are easier to follow than those delivered by some of the researchers and are more focused on the kind of things that will come up in the exam. These student tutors are very popular.

Medical School B has a philosophy that emphasises learning over teaching and that students must learn to become life-long learners, with excellent skills in working out what they need to know, learning what they need to and applying this learning to improving patient care. Binge superficial learning for exams is to be discouraged. Their curriculum in the first few years uses PBL (problem-based learning) or case-based learning, lots of facilitation and few lectures. The library is busy and students are probably expected to keep some kind of portfolio that encourages them to learn continuously. The school tries to keep focus away from the exams, which generally ask for application and problem solving, focusing on patient care.

This medical school deliberately leaves students feeling a little anxious, leaving some questions open in their minds to encourage them to be puzzled and want to look things up. The school exhibits 'paradoxical paternalism' in that it tries to encourage the students to become more independent, not to need its teaching and encouragement. The students get stressed in the second half of the year about the exams and a group of senior students start revision lectures. These are much more focused on the kind of things that will come up in the exam and claim to teach the junior students exactly what they need to know, so they do not need to do any bookwork at all. These student tutors are very popular.

In Medical School A, the student tutors teach in a way that is consistent with the curriculum and are likely to do little harm. In Medical School B, the student tutors are unintentionally sabotaging the key message that the School wants students to learn – that *they* are responsible for their learning, not some outside source and that cramming for exams is bad, the focus should be on learning for patient care.

Semi-formal peer tutoring can, therefore, have unexpected and sometimes unwanted outcomes in terms of student learning. Your medical school will have some talented educationalists (sometimes somewhere obvious, sometimes tucked away somewhere) who can help you consider wider implications of peer teaching programmes, if that is something that you would like to set up?

Mentoring and coaching

'*Mentoring is increasingly viewed as a key factor contributing to a successful career in medicine*'

Dimitriadis *et al.*, 2012

Some famous mentoring relationships:

- Socrates to Plato
- John Stevens Henslow (academic and clergyman) to Charles Darwin
- Mariah Carey to Christina Aguilera
- Elmore Leonard (crime writer) to Quentin Tarantino
- Maya Angelou to Oprah Winfrey
- Dadabhai Naoroji (Indian leader) to Gandhi.

Mentoring is a natural human activity that has been around since the ancient Greeks (Garvey and Langridge, 2003) and is an effective way of learning and developing. Most medical schools in the United Kingdom, however, do not have formal mentoring schemes, so it may be a good idea to set something up for yourself, especially as we know that medical students who have a mentor perform better academically (Dimitriadis *et al.*, 2012).

This section will look at both sides of mentoring, at being a mentor and a mentee, as both roles have benefits.

What is mentoring?

You could be forgiven for not *quite* understanding what mentoring and coaching are, as these terms are often used interchangeably and can mean different things in different contexts. For the purposes of this chapter, however, we will accept that mentoring is:

- a one-to-one relationship with someone who is either more experienced or senior or it can also be a relationship between equals, the primary aim of which is to help the mentee to see things in a new way, learn new ways of doing things and see new possibilities by offering support and advice to help the mentee reach their aims.
- In contrast, coaching tends to have a specific goal; for example, helping someone to prepare to present a patient, or a paper at a conference or a dissertation. Coaching can be one-to-one or in a small group and can be a relationship between equals or between senior and junior.

Finding the right mentor

So a mentor/coach can be:

- A peer
- Someone in the year(s) above you/or on another course/in another medical school
- Someone you know well
- Someone you do not know at all
- An official or an unofficial arrangement.

But, finding a *suitable* mentor is important as the literature suggests that a mentor who is 'found' or identified by the mentee tends to lead to a more successful relationship (Huskins *et al.*, 2011). Of course, the topics and issues you want to work on may suggest the mentor/coach you want to work with. Ask yourself some questions first:

- Who has expertise in the topic I want to work on?
- Who operates/learns/achieves in a way I respect?
- Do I want to work with a peer or someone with more experienced than me?
- Who do I respect to be honest and have my best interests at heart?
- Should I work with a group of people instead of one?
- Who will I get on with?
- Who can recommend a mentor/coach for me?
- Has anyone had prior mentoring/coaching experience?

Of course, it will be important to work with a range of mentors/coaches over time as each will bring a different style, strength or expertise, but the important unifying factor in all mentoring/coaching arrangements is that the mentee is an active participant in the relationship, selecting the mentor/coach, arranging the meetings and deciding on the topics/issues to discuss. Mentoring is in effect an active process that brings about active change.

> *I started a group with two other people in my year to prepare for an important presentation for our research project. The others weren't fussed at first, but agreed later that it was really useful and gave us the confidence to know that we had covered everything.*
>
> Nasreen, fourth-year student.

Being a mentor and finding the right mentee

Becoming a mentor or coach can be a really positive experience that brings rewards. It will help you to expand and improve your ability to work with others, develop skills of facilitation and exploration rather than just giving advice, will give you a wider perspective on medicine and learning in general, will increase your powers of reflection and it can be personally satisfying to help someone achieve a goal or aim.

To identify whether you have got what it takes to be a mentor and also find a suitable mentee, you will also need to ask yourself some questions:

- Is there any kind of training available in mentoring/coaching I can sign up for?
- What topics/areas do I have some expertise in?
- Am I encouraging and empathic?
- Do I have an open mind and a flexible attitude to people?

- Do I have the time to mentor someone?
- Do I know someone who has already been a mentor?
- Is there someone I can talk to about mentoring in my medical school?
- What kind of mentee do I want to work with?
- Do I want to work with someone more junior or a peer?
- Should I work with a group of people or just one?
- Who do I usually get on with?

As a mentor/coach, it will be important to have someone you can talk to in case you need advice or help with a particular situation. This could be a tutor, other mentors, student welfare officer or counselling service. Identifying this person in advance is a good idea so that you have a clear idea of your boundaries and know when and where you can go for support or advice (Garvey and Langridge, 2003). Success in mentoring is not only knowing what it can be used for, but also knowing when someone needs more help than a mentoring arrangement can offer.

What to work on in a mentoring/coaching arrangement

We know from the literature and from personal experience that it is vital to align your personal expectations with those of the mentor/mentee. These should be negotiated in advance of setting things up as they require a clear idea of what is to be achieved. If you as the mentee have only a vague notion that you 'want to become a better medical student', then it is time to do some work on yourself and be far less vague! What would help you become a better student; is it better study skills, better time management, better working with patients, better group work ability etc.? The mentees have to develop insight into their own strengths and weaknesses by being analytical. Remember, mentoring is about being an active participant in any arrangement, not expecting extra teaching or for the mentor/coach to sort your life out in some way. Here are some ideas for topics, but you will have many of your own:

- Effective studying
- Peer tutoring
- Exam techniques
- Time management/life-work balance
- Working on the ward/clinic/surgery
- Conversational English/written English
- Working with patients
- Understanding the medical school or hospital culture
- Presenting patients/papers/posters
- Doing research/audit.

Chapter 12

I found having a mentor really, really helpful. It was better than asking a tutor for help as my mentor understood where I was coming from and understood the difficulties I was having.

Dan, second-year graduate student.

Using a mentoring model

Many models exist, but we offer one here that is an amalgamation of several models that we think covers most things for the mentee/mentor.

Step one – for the mentee – analysing what you need

Clarify your strengths and weaknesses.
    Identify your knowledge and skills gaps; are they

- Personal
- Professional development
- Skill development
- Study guidance
- Research.

Step one – for the mentor – analysing what you need

Clarify your strengths and weaknesses.
Have you set aside time for mentoring?
Have you had training/talked to other mentors?
Where can you go for advice and support?

Step two – identify a mentor/mentee

Peer or senior?
Group or individual?
Known or unknown?
Who can recommend a mentor/mentee?
Have they had any experience of mentoring already?

Step three – the first meeting, setting up rules of engagement

Share your background, values and expectations of each other.
Agree on what you want to work on.
Agree on how many times you will meet, for how long, dates, times, locations and so on.
Agree on rules; for example, turning up on time, preparing for meetings, completing tasks and so on.

Step four – developing the relationship

Set goals and expectations.

Ask questions.

Listen.

Complete any tasks agreed on.

Ask for/give feedback.

Respond and be flexible.

Set agendas for each meeting.

Look at any progress made.

Step five – ending the arrangement and moving on

Talk about when the arrangement should end.

Talk about next steps.

What has been achieved?

Think about future mentoring opportunities.

Adapted from Alred *et al.* (2003) and Zerzan *et al.* (2009).

A word about peer coaching

Some people work very well in peer pairs or triads to work on particular problems or prepare for events like exams or OSCEs (Objective Structured Clinical Examinations). Many of the issues we have already covered apply here, such as agreeing on topics to work on, setting up a schedule, group rules and completing tasks on time. This type of coaching works well for specific events, but does not tend to deal in any depth with more personal goals. Setting up a group such as this is a very successful way to prepare for learning challenges ahead, and remember, you do not have to work with friends in this kind of arrangement, pick people you respect or who work in a way that is successful.

Case study

Roberto

Roberto joined the medical school in the third year having studied in his home country for his early years in medicine. Coming to the United Kingdom and starting a new course at the same time was traumatic and he found that 4 months in he still did not have many friends in his year, his English was not as fluent as he would have liked, particularly when talking to patients and his mock OSCE results were not good for clinical communication.

He had good memories of a mentoring arrangement at his last college and set about finding a mentor to help him. He found Kai who was 2 years ahead

Chapter 12

of him and who was also an international student, although from a different country, and who was not only doing well in OSCEs but also really enjoyed meeting and clerking patients.

They agreed to meet on six occasions to work on conversational English, talking and clerking patients on the wards and integrating into the year. Kai pointed Roberto in the direction of an advanced spoken English class run by the local council and introduced him to a voluntary club run by the Student Union for children with intellectual disabilities, where he volunteered to work once a week. He also went with Roberto twice on his clinical placement to clerk patients on the wards in pairs, which both found really useful. Although Kai was 2 years ahead in his clinical knowledge, Roberto found some of the social skills he used with patients to be really useful and hearing his advanced clinical questions and reasoning really helped him to understand why some questions were asked. They gave each other feedback on their communication with patients, which was mutually helpful.

Over time, with the volunteering work and spoken language classes, Roberto's English as well as his confidence improved and he started to join in with more Student Union events. He set a target of clerking and examining five patients each week as well as grabbing every opportunity he could to talk to patients informally. He passed his OSCE well and had some friends to go about with by the end of the year.

Kai was pleased to have helped and had enjoyed their paired clerking. He felt he had used his experience of being an international student to good effect and added mentoring to his CV.

References and further reading

Teaching references

Ertmer, P. A. & Newby, T. J. (1993). Behaviorism, cognitivism, constructivism: Comparing critical features from an instructional design perspective. *Performance Improvement Quarterly*, 6(4), 50–72.

Gagne, R. M. (1985). *The Conditions of Learning and Theory of Instruction*. 4th edn. New York; London, Holt, Rinehart and Winston.

O'Connor, H. M. (2002). Training undergraduate medical students in procedural skills. *Emergency Medicine (Fremantle)*, 14(2), 131–135.

Further reading around teaching

Cantillon, P. & Wood, D. (2010). *ABC of Learning and Teaching in Medicine*. 2nd edn. Chichester, Wiley-Blackwell.

Jarvis, P., Holford, J. & Griffin, C. (2003). *The Theory & Practice of Learning*. 2nd edn. London, Kogan Page.

Mentoring and coaching

Alred, G., Garvey, B. & Smith, R. (2003). *The Mentoring Pocketbook*. Hampshire, Management Pocketbooks Ltd.

Dimitriadis, K., von der Borch, P., Stormann, S., Meinel, F. G., Moder, S., Reincke, M. & Fischer, M. R. (2012). Characteristics of mentoring relationships formed by medical students and faculty. *Medical Education Online*, *17*, 17242.

Garvey, B. & Langridge, K. (2003). *Mentoring in Schools Pocketbook*. Hampshire, Teacher's Pocketbooks.

Huskins, W. C., Silet, K., Weber-Main, A. M., Begg, M. D., Fowler, V. G., Jr., Hamilton, J. & Fleming, M. (2011). Identifying and aligning expectations in a mentoring relationship. *Clinical and Translational Science*, *4*(6), 439–447.

Zerzan, J. T., Hess, R., Schur, E., Phillips, R. S. & Rigotti, N. (2009). Making the most of mentors: a guide for mentees. *Academic Medicine*, *84*(1), 140–144.

Questions and answers

Q: What is the difference between the revision lectures on anatomy we receive and setting up a peer coaching group to review anatomy learning?

A: Revision lectures are important and are a good way of reviewing and consolidating what you know – they are a great way of brushing up your knowledge. However, they can be quite passive and it can be difficult to know how to apply this knowledge to, say, your clinical skills and clinical reasoning. Setting up a peer coaching group, however, allows you to operationalise your knowledge and try things out with others to embed your knowledge into authentic practice and therefore into deep learning.

Finding out what a cruciate ligament looks like, feels like, moves like and what it stops you from doing when damaged, will become more real in a peer coaching group.

Q: I tend to be the sort of person who likes to be taught things and in turn I like to give learners a thorough overview of a subject when I teach them. Should I be doing more than this?

A: It depends on the type of teacher you want to be! Knowing and giving lots of information about the subject you are teaching is helpful, but is really just the beginning. Getting your learners actively engaged in the subject, questioning things, trying things out, reading around the literature, arguing with you, all helps them to embed the subject into deep learning and is therefore much more likely to be remembered and acted upon.

Q: I have not got a lot of interest in teaching clinical skills, but I hear that it is a great way to meet girls.

A: Get reading the chapter on professionalism!

Chapter 12

Chapter 13 **Professionalism: not as straightforward as you think**

OVERVIEW

This whole book is about professionalism – about striving to do your best for patient care: professionalism is simple. This chapter specifically focuses on how to learn professionalism, including how it is assessed. Fundamentally this chapter highlights that professionalism is far from simple and, we hope, will give you a deeper awareness of the challenges around maintaining professionalism.

Introduction

Few people will tell you this, but professionalism is a fuzzy concept. Do not get us wrong, some behaviours are absolutely, incontrovertibly unprofessional – steal from the hospital, cheat in your exams, turn up to the wards under the influence of alcohol or recreational drugs; everyone would agree that these are unprofessional behaviours. Similarly, there are a whole range of clearly professional behaviours. There is, however, a really messy area in between. This chapter does not aim to tell you how to behave professionally, we imagine that you should be able to spot the obviously unprofessional behaviours yourself, instead we aim to explore the messy areas. Have a look at the following questions and grade each one 'clearly OK', 'clearly unprofessional' or 'messy'.

How to Succeed at Medical School: An Essential Guide to Learning, Second Edition.
Dason Evans and Jo Brown.
© 2015 John Wiley & Sons, Ltd. Published 2015 by John Wiley & Sons, Ltd.

A medical student drinks too much at a party and has a hangover the next day.

A first-year medical student drinks too much at a party and has a hangover the next day; he or she turns up to lectures but finds it hard to concentrate. He or she has to leave to vomit.

A third-year medical student drinks too much at a party and has a hangover the next day; he or she turns up to assist in the operating theatre but finds it hard to concentrate. He or she has to leave to vomit.

A foundation-year doctor (Intern) drinks too much at a party and has a hangover the next day; he or she turns up to assist in the operating theatre but finds it hard to concentrate. He or she has to leave to vomit.

---

1 A first-year medical student thinks that homosexuality is morally wrong. He or she makes every effort to ensure that this does not affect how he or she approaches patients and colleagues who are homosexual.

2 A fourth-year medical student used to be quite homophobic. When he or she was at school, he or she tweeted a highly witty and profoundly inappropriate homophobic comment, which was then re-tweeted widely. He or she regrets this.

3 A fourth-year medical student thinks that homosexuality is morally wrong. He or she makes every effort to ensure that this does not affect how he or she approaches patients and colleagues who are homosexual. He or she re-tweets a highly witty and profoundly inappropriate homophobic comment to a friend.

A doctor steals morphine from the drug cupboard in the hospital.

A doctor takes two paracetamol from the drug cupboard in the hospital.

A doctor steals the latest TV series DVD box set from a shop.

A doctor downloads the latest TV series through a peer-to-peer file-sharing website.

A doctor gives his or her brother his or her entire MP3 music collection on a memory stick.

Chapter 13

There are some general principles that run through this chapter. Firstly, that there are absolute extremes of 'clearly unprofessional' and 'clearly professional', but things are less clear in between these extremes and, indeed, it is also not clear if there might be a category of 'exemplary professionalism' above 'clearly professional'. Models of professionalism are sometimes binary and sometimes a longitudinal scale. Definitions of professionalism are not absolutely fixed – they vary over time, geography and generations. Perhaps worryingly, your professionalism will not be judged by your peers but rather those probably two generations above you.

As a medical student, you are learning medical professionalism at the same time as you are learning everything else and you will be assessed on your professionalism, just as you will be assessed on your other competencies. You will be expected to develop professionalism on a trajectory from year one until graduation and beyond, as a gradual transition (through 'proto-professionalism') as you progress through the course.

The Internet, in general, and social media, specifically, form a professionalism minefield. You should actively manage your digital footprint and assume that anything that you put on social media, however 'secure' your privacy settings, will be seen by your mother, the dean of the medical school and everyone in between.

As with most book chapters on professionalism, we provide some reminders about patient confidentiality and, unlike most, we discuss sexual attraction within the confines of professional behaviour!

This is not a definitive chapter on professionalism and we just hope that this chapter will make you think, help you spot possible pitfalls and that it might trigger your curiosity. We hope that it encourages you to read the suggested reading at the end of the chapter and maybe even read a little further afield, perhaps starting a debating group or looking at your institutions policies and practices and whether they are keeping up with the rapidly changing electronic landscape.

What is professionalism?

Definitions of professionalism

In the United Kingdom, fundamental issues of medical professionalism are defined by the UK's General Medical Council (GMC), principally but not exclusively by their booklet *Good Medical Practice* which is regularly updated and available on the GMC website, www.gmc-uk.org. Within this chapter, we refer to the version published in March 2013 and updated in April 2014. This booklet is available as a PDF for free on the website, as well as in hard copy. It includes a summary in the form of 'duties of a doctor' as listed in the following section.

The duties of a doctor registered with the General Medical Council

Patients must be able to trust doctors with their lives and health. To justify that trust you must show respect for human life and make sure your practice meets the standards expected of you in four domains.

Knowledge, skills and performance
- Make the care of your patient your first concern.
- Provide a good standard of practice and care.
  - Keep your professional knowledge and skills up to date.
  - Recognise and work within the limits of your competence.

Safety and quality
- Take prompt action if you think that patient safety, dignity or comfort is being compromised.
- Protect and promote the health of patients and the public.

Communication, partnership and teamwork
- Treat patients as individuals and respect their dignity.
  - Treat patients politely and considerately.
  - Respect patients' right to confidentiality.
- Work in partnership with patients.
  - Listen to, and respond to, their concerns and preferences.
  - Give patients the information they want or need in a way they can understand.
  - Respect patients' right to reach decisions with you about their treatment and care.
  - Support patients in caring for themselves to improve and maintain their health.
  - Work with colleagues in the ways that best serve patients' interests.

Maintaining trust
- Be honest and open and act with integrity.
- Never discriminate unfairly against patients or colleagues.
- Never abuse your patients' trust in you or the public's trust in the profession.

You are personally accountable for your professional practice and must always be prepared to justify your decisions and actions.

Chapter 13

We would highly recommend that you read the full document and consider how it relates to you. You may wish to re-read it on a regular basis and keep up with any changes.

There are multiple other definitions of professionalism, ranging from ones that require extensive *judgement*, through to detailed lists. One definition that we rather like is from Herbert Swick, based in Montana, USA, who developed a 'normative definition of medical professionalism', which combines many features found in other definitions:

Toward a Normative Definition of Medical Professionalism

Herbert M. Swick, MD (2000).

Acad. Med, 612–616.

1 Physicians subordinate their own interests to the interests of others.

2 Physicians adhere to high ethical and moral standards.

3 Physicians respond to societal needs and their behaviours reflect a social contract with the communities served.

4 Physicians evince core humanistic values, including honesty and integrity, caring and compassion, altruism and empathy, respect for others and trust-worthiness.

5 Physicians exercise accountability for themselves and for their colleagues.

6 Physicians demonstrate a continuing commitment to excellence.

7 Physicians exhibit a commitment to scholarship and to advancing their field.

8 Physicians deal with high levels of complexity and uncertainty.

9 Physicians reflect upon their actions and decisions.

Putting 'professionalism' into PubMed will find you a huge number of different concepts and definitions of professionalism from around the world. Most of them have similar core principles.

Past present and future

The concept of medical professionalism and its assessment has changed markedly over the last 50 years. Shifting from a poorly defined impression, paralleled by Justice Potter Stewart's definition of obscenity ('I know it when I see it', 1964) through to a host of definitions based around attitudes and specific behaviours (such as those listed by the GMC and Dr Swick). These definitions tend to see professionalism as an all or nothing (good enough) concept. Either a doctor is honest or not, there are no degrees of honesty.

There are two problems with this 'trait' approach to defining professionalism. Firstly, there is a question about 'people' versus 'behaviours' – can a usually professional person have a momentary unprofessional lapse? Does this make them 'unprofessional'? Could an unprofessional behaviour be exhibited by a professional person? Secondly, there has been a shift to thinking of professionalism as a continuum, with the learning of professionalism representing a longitudinal developmental process. Sean Hilton and Henry Slotnick (2005) coined the term 'proto-professionalism'. By this, they mean the early stages of development of professionalism. Implicit in their theory is that professionalism can be learnt and that curricula should be created that 'foster the acquisition and maintenance of professionalism'; they highlight how 'Adverse environmental conditions in the hidden curriculum may have powerful [negative] effects'. The GMC have published specific guidance for medical students – 'Medical students: professional values and fitness to practise' – again, something worth finding on their website and having a read of.

Over time, therefore, concepts of professionalism have shifted from the individual themselves to the behaviours that they exhibit, from simple binary concepts to a continuum and from a trait that someone does or does not have to something that can be learnt. Not only do concepts of professionalism vary over time, but also by geography, culture and context. To quote a friend and colleague who is a doctor and educator in Pakistan: '*I think it might be greatly affected by the surrounding environment where that profession is being practiced. Ethics, resourcefulness, altruism and the will to practice to the highest standards will always be integral to it.*' – Dr Syed Asghar Naqi (2014).

Patients above all …

All concepts of professionalism put the patient central to what it is to be a doctor. Put patients first. This is not as straightforward as it might seem. Indeed, there is good research evidence that altruism falls and cynicism climbs as students progress through medical school. No one is quite sure why this is; however, we can hypothesise that this occurs as an unconscious drift, starting perhaps with side effects of assessment and then progressing in the clinical years through negative role modelling.

Assessment drives learning. This is a depressing but unfortunately true statement. First-year medical students arrive keen to learn for patient care and pretty quickly the curriculum shifts them into focusing their learning for exams. Strategic learning is common, perhaps essential at medical school; however, it becomes increasingly easy to lose sight of the patient in the process.

Case studies

- A colleague trained some years ago in a medical school where he knew that, in the essay-based anatomy exam, he would have to choose to write four out of five possible essays. He deliberately and strategically chose not to learn the anatomy of the leg, but spent that saved time on extra learning

Chapter 13

for the anatomy of the other systems. He strategically decided that he just would not answer the question on the leg. Similarly, and depressingly up to date, in 2009, Ben Wormold (who was a medical student at the time) showed rather elegantly that when anatomy score was poorly weighted and had a low contribution to the end of year exams that medical students spent less time learning it, despite fully and consciously acknowledging that anatomy knowledge was essential to practice as a doctor. When the weighting increased, students spent more time learning it.

- We ran some training for final-year students on acute confusional state. It is very common for junior doctors to be called to a patient who is confused and asked to assess them and institute treatment. It is quite possible to make things much worse through the wrong management (e.g. by using benzodiazepines for sedation), or to miss an important cause, with potentially drastic consequences (e.g. missing hypoxia). Despite acknowledging that managing patients with acute confusional state was a bread-and-butter task for new doctors, and also that it had been poorly covered previously in their teaching, these students were not interested in the session at all. They were worried about their forthcoming OSCE (Objective Structured Clinical Examination) and knew that it would be very difficult to have a station on acute confusional state.

- Books that promise to help you pass exams 'at a glance', 'easy guide to passing exams', 'idiots guides' and so on are increasingly common in medical bookshops. They generally promise to help you pass exams with the minimum of effort. Why would someone who puts patient care first buy only such books? Surely, they would want to work hard for a deep understanding? OK, in order to make a point, we are being a little harsh on some of these books and they can often be useful to give an overview of a topic before delving deeper using thicker books (Chapter 2), and for clinical skills OSCE books can play a role in helping structure feedback ('the checklist' – see Chapter 3); however, we would like you to reflect on how these titles may unconsciously shift your focus from patients to exams

Role models have an amazingly powerful role to play in learning. We probably learn professionalism, professional identity and professional behaviours largely through role models. Unfortunately, these lessons are not always positive ones and you can find yourself soaking up cynicism from negative role models. Imagine that a popular and entertaining junior doctor introduces you to the game of 'TURF the patient' where he tries to reduce his workload by finding reasons to transfer his team's patients to other teams. He convinces the gynaecologists to take the woman with abdominal pain who might have appendicitis, the rheumatologists to take the patient with diverticulitis because she also has severe spinal arthritis and is working on getting an elderly woman with abdominal pain taken by the elderly care doctors. At some point, the 'game' has taken over and become an end point in itself, rather than truly trying to do the best for each patient.

So, if the primacy of patient care can be easily forgotten, thanks to the unintended messages in the curricula and assessments at your medical school and thanks to the culture and charismatic role models that you may come across, what can you do to ensure patient care remains foremost in your mind? We think the solution is simple:

- Go back to Chapter 1 and go through the section on *What Motivates You* again. Think also about how you would have answered this before you arrived at medical school. See if you can dig out your medical school application and the personal statement that you wrote. We somehow doubt that you joined medical school because you wanted to pass exams for the rest of your life.
- Find a definition of professionalism, or even what it is to be a doctor, that you like, that you can identify with. If you do not like the GMC's version or Dr Swick's or any of the host of others, write your own. Perhaps along the lines of 'I study at medical school because I want to become a doctor. I want to become a doctor who … /because … ; I therefore study at medical school to … '
- Consider a way of reminding yourself of this throughout your training – perhaps an automated e-mail, a diary reminder, an image as a desktop background, your phone home screen, or something as low tech as a sheet of paper stuck to your wall.
- Consider how you can embed this belief into how you learn and into your daily routine.

Professionalism within the school and hospital

Here, professionalism is relatively easy to define. There is gross unprofessionalism and then niggling unprofessionalism. Gross unprofessionalism includes stealing, cheating, lying and so forth. There would be little debate if you asked anyone if a medical student who cheats in his exams should be allowed to become a doctor. More niggling issues include dress, punctuality, conduct, attitude and so forth. At what point does the student who is frequently late become unprofessional? What about the student with inappropriate clothing? Or a student with bright pink hair?

It is worthwhile highlighting that your professionalism will not be judged by your peers, but rather by a different generation. You may feel that some aspects of dress, even the language that you use are appropriate for your generation; however, you should ensure that they are seen as appropriate for the generation of patients that you are caring for and the advanced years of those that will be judging you. We talk more about this when we discuss social media and also the assessment of professionalism.

Breaking patient confidentiality is an area of gross unprofessionalism that can easily catch students out. Rules around patient confidentiality are very clear. Any notes that you make and take away must be anonymised in such a way that the patient is not identifiable. This is fairly obvious. Trickier are the conversations that you will have with peers and loved ones. Doctors are story-tellers, we use case histories and stories about our experiences to pass on learning, it is both important for learning and also innate within the culture of what it is to be a doctor. Be cautious about who you tell these stories to (remember that those outside of medicine may not have the same understanding of confidentiality as you do) and be exceptionally careful about unintended audiences – restaurants, coffee shops, lifts and public transport are common and yet entirely inappropriate places to discuss any form of patient information. Even if you change the details to anonymise the case, someone overhearing may think that you are breaching confidentiality, breaching the trust that they have in the profession.

In terms of confidentiality, data protection and professionalism, in general, it is NEVER appropriate for a medical student to take photographs of a patient, regardless of the intention behind doing so. Such a seemingly innocuous activity (even presidents and prime-ministers seem to take 'selfies' on their phones) is riddled with ethical challenges: we have listed a few, but by no means all of them, below:

- Consent: most likely you have not been trained to ask for formal consent as a medical student (apart from consent to learn). How will you ensure that both the notes (patient record) and the patient have a copy of the consent and that somehow the picture will be linked with the consent, while maintaining patient confidentiality? What do you include in the consent? Blanket 'use this picture for anything' is almost certainly not something that a patient can truly give informed consent to. Patients have the right to withdraw consent – how would they do that? If a digital image has circulated, how can you remove it from circulation?
- Ease of errors: most of us now synchronise our pictures across devices. How can you maintain security? What if you take a picture on your phone of a patient's venous leg ulcer; you intend to print it at the top of your personal notes as a hook to hang your learning on and then delete the digital image, the patient gives her willing consent for this. Unfortunately, your young brother finds it on the tablet at home, or the cache on your computer and puts it on Facebook with the comments 'Ew Gross! Never wanna be a

doctor'; it goes viral, the patient and her family are mortified. If you think this is farfetched, consider for a moment how many people you know who have had their social media and/or e-mail hacked, or even hijacked by a friend or family member who they thought was trustworthy/responsible but was not.

- Data protection: there are laws governing data privacy. Photographs tend to have to adhere to higher levels of the law, as 'sensitive' data can be inferred from them (such as ethnicity). Furthermore, synchronising your photos or even e-mailing them almost always passes your data through servers that are outside the European Union and so must adhere to even more stringent laws about data export. The law is far behind the technology.

- Professional guidance: there are various documents on the GMC website that are relevant, including 'Making and using visual and audio recordings of patients'.

Professionalism outside of the 'workplace'

Probably the most fascinating and messy aspect of professionalism is the role that a doctor's behaviour outside the workplace plays in the judgement of his or her professionalism as a doctor. A doctor must, for example, inform the GMC if they have had any convictions or cautions by the police, including road traffic offences. Whatever you think about it, the GMC expects doctors to be professional not only at work, but also out of work. This includes 'the protection of patients, maintenance of public confidence in the profession and the declaring and upholding of proper standards of conduct and behaviour'. Duties of a doctor state that 'You must make sure that your conduct at all times justifies your patients' trust in you and the public's trust in the profession.'

Medical students are in a transition between lay people and professionals. One aspect of this transmission is characterised by the development of professionalism (Sean Hilton's 'proto-professionalism'). The expected standard of behaviour of a medical student, therefore, reflects the level of their training. This includes their behaviour outside of the 'workplace', whether that be in the park, the pub, the road or on the Internet. The specific GMC guidance states that '*Students must be aware that their behaviour outside the clinical environment, including in their personal lives, may have an impact on their fitness to practise […]. Their behaviour at all times must justify the trust the public places in the medical profession.*'

Social media, your digital footprint and professionalism

Social media is likely to fundamentally change the way that we think about professionalism and the crossover between work life and home life for professionals. Unfortunately, this change is unlikely to happen quickly. For the first time in history, every single conversation can be recorded indelibly. A flippant comment, a whinge about a bad day at work or a piece of information about a patient that you retrospectively feel you could have anonymised better: all these will be indelible. While you may believe that you are having an informal conversation with friends, you are, in fact, producing a written publication that will never be deleted.

Challenges to your online privacy may occur because of changes in the past, present or future.

- In the past, changing your e-mail address may lose you access to your history and to control over privacy settings.
- In the present, privacy rules keep changing and will continue to change, with privacy (or at least Internet privacy) becoming an 'outdated concept'. Unfortunately, those judging you on your online professionalism tend to be of a generation that may find it difficult to keep up or even understand the shifting culture created by social media, apps currently take your address book and suggest people that you know; if you give a patient your e-mail address, they may gain easy access to your profiles (Google, Tumblr, Facebook etc.). Hackers and 'friends' who get onto your profile can cause no end of grief and it is difficult to prove that it was not you when an inappropriate post contains your 'digital signature'.
- In the future, more challenges are on their way. As companies buy each other and merge, your digital footprints can be merged. 'Big data' will bring its own challenges and facial recognition is becoming excellent, it will not be long until all the pictures of you on the Internet are searchable, whether you put them on, or some random tourist took a picture of you vomiting on a stag night.

In April 2013, Britain's first youth crime commissioner resigned from her post less than a week after her appointment. Paris Brown was 17 at the time and resigned because of inappropriate tweets that she sent when she was between the ages of 14 and 16. The police and crime commissioner who appointed her said 'I think it would have been absolutely impossible to have found a young person who had not made a silly, foolish or even perhaps a deeply offensive comment during their short lifetime. I'm sure everyone has said or written something they regret – I certainly have. Unfortunately, today we live in an Internet world where many people air their views in the public domain.'

So what can you do?

- Clean up your online profile as much as you can, go back as far as you can and remember social media platforms that you might have used some years ago.
- Ensure that your privacy settings are as high as they can be, restrict your friends' lists to people that you know.
- Never put *anything* (text, pictures, sharing others' posts) on the Internet, either in the public OR private domain, that you would not want your mother to see (or for that matter your dean, medical regulator, future boss).
- Social media can provide great support networks, but if people in your network start acting unprofessionally, tell them gently and if things do not change, leave that group, just as you would do if your colleagues were acting unprofessionally in the coffee shop in the hospital.
- See if your medical school has a specialist in e-professionalism and start an open discussion, engage with the published literature (see *Recommended Reading*).
- Bernadette John is one such person and states that 'The landscape has totally changed, and social [media] cannot be ignored any more – we all have a footprint, we need to consciously be architects of our profiles, online and off.'
- In a faculty development workshop for GPs recently, Julian Sheather, Deputy Head of Ethics at the British Medical Association, gave a useful analogy to driving a car: before heading off you check the mirrors, put on your seatbelt, check it is out of gear before starting – basic safety measures that you do when about to drive a car. He argued that using social media should be no different. You avoid driving when your judgment is impaired from alcohol, you should avoid the Internet too.

The RCGP 'Social Media Highway Code' is currently one of the best resources for doctors and medical students to learn how to effectively manage their digital footprint (see *Recommended Reading*).

Sexual and professional boundaries

One of the authors (Dason Evans) worked on another book where students, staff and others suggested things that medical students could do in spare moments on the wards (see *Recommended Reading*). We clustered the submissions into themes and drafted a commentary around these themes. One theme was around sexualised comments. Nothing too risqué, principally comments around ranking the attractiveness of the team members or flirting with members of the multi-disciplinary team, certainly nothing that we would class as 'unprofessional'.

The reviewers of the draft version of the book were uncomfortable with the quotes and wanted them taken out, but liked the surrounding commentary

Chapter 13

that highlighted that doctors (and, indeed, medical students) were human. We found this fascinating that the commentary was valued, but quotes that validated the commentary were not; perhaps they were too close to reality.

Medical students and doctors of all ages have sexual desires. They sometimes find each other attractive and occasionally may find patients attractive too. Despite this, and rather strangely, the topic of doctors being sexual beings is a taboo, it is rarely spoken about, apart from in cases of misconduct. Apparently, it is shocking that doctors are human. The whole topic of sexual boundaries for doctors is very interesting and we have included some further, recommended reading at the end of the chapter. The simple take-home message, however, is that it is NEVER appropriate to have an intimate relationship with a patient. It is important not to lose this message when looking at some of the less clear aspects.

Professional boundaries and power imbalances

It is inappropriate for a doctor to have an intimate relationship with a patient; this is very clearly stated by the GMC in its guidance on intimate relationships – it is covered both in *Good Medical Practice* and in supplementary advice – *Maintaining Boundaries,* both available from www.gmc-uk.org. There have been some very high profile cases (e.g. Kerr/Haslam, Peter Green, Clifford Ayling enquiries) and we would recommend that you look up the summaries of these cases, which are readily available on the Internet.

From time to time you will, of course, find a patient attractive, from time to time a patient may find you attractive and occasionally you will find each other attractive. This is all normal and human. The wrongness is when you act on it. It is wrong for a number of reasons: there is a power imbalance that may make it difficult all round; the relationship that you have been forming is not a normal relationship, it is a doctor–patient relationship – the patient sees a doctor, gives respect, may value your guidance and they may well confuse the fact that you care *about* what happens to them with that you care *for* them; there are often aspects of vulnerability to the patient and their relationship to you. Sometimes aspects of the doctor–patient relationship including sharing of secrets, assurances of confidentiality, empathy and compassion can resemble aspects of an intimate relationship (while being entirely different). This can lead to confusion not only for the patient, but also for you as the professional. Talking through your feelings with someone neutral and wise will allow you to rationalise what is happening and manage it professionally and appropriately. Desire is ubiquitous and yet managing desire is a part of professionalism that is rarely discussed.

An intimate relationship between a doctor and their patient is wrong. We would imagine that for similar reasons, a relationship between a patient and their medical student would be wrong too. What do you think about other relationships based on trust, power imbalance and dependence? What about a consultant asking a medical student out, a lecturer (or dean even) asking a junior student out, or even a final-year student asking a first-year out in fresher's week? What are your personal boundaries? For example, when you are a junior doctor, an impressionable first-year student asks you out because 'it must be just so amazing to be a doctor', what would you do? Do you think what is right for you is the same as what is right for all your peers?

Assessment of professionalism at Medical School

'Moral panic' is a sociological term describing a chain of actions that starts with an event that causes concern and threatens established norms. This usually results in hostility towards a given group that spreads and gains consensus, usually through news services. Following this, there is a disproportionate response, which often does not address the initial event and then concerns move on and away.

There have been two highly influential events resulting in the assessment of professionalism at Medical School. This first was Harold Shipman, a trusted GP who was found to be a serial killer, arrested in September 1998 and subsequently proven guilty of 15 murders and suspected to have murdered up to 250 others. He murdered his patients, shocking the nation at such a betrayal of trust in a professional. Something had to be done and this cascaded down to medical schools needing to spot 'bad apples' – not just assessing knowledge and skills but also professionalism.

The second influential event was a paper by Maxine Papadakis and colleagues in 2004. She conducted a retrospective case control study looking at doctors who trained in one medical school who had been disciplined by the medical board of California over 10 years (68 doctors). She found that those who ran into trouble later were roughly twice as likely to have had professionalism issues at medical school than matched controls. She is a great speaker and well worth attending if you see her headlining at a conference. She is always quick to point out that her study was retrospective in nature and that she did not explore how strong a predictor unprofessional behaviour at medical school was on future unprofessional behaviour. All the same, it appeared as a result, reasonable to assess medical students' professionalism as with any other competency.

There are various different methods used for assessing professionalism. They usually rely on multiple judgements or reports, sometimes formalised (such as the consultant on any attachment that you are on filling out a form), sometimes ad hoc (you swear at the librarian for giving you a fine, he fills out a professionalism report form) and often a combination of both. Occasionally, there are more formal assessments around professionalism such as OSCE stations or multiple-choice questions (including the SJT or situational judgement test – see Chapters 10 and 11), although these are often seen as being a little too distant from real life.

Every medical school has its own professionalism assessment and different plan on how to deal with issues that arise. In general, a single big issue will usually result in some sort of professional conduct committee, which will investigate, meet with the student and come up with a plan. Steal drugs from the hospital and you are likely to be removed from medical training permanently and reported to the police. Smaller issues in a junior medical student are usually seen as an opportunity for learning. Refuse to pay your library fine and you will be asked to pay, apologise and do some kind of assignment to help you consider the professionalism implications. Repeated smaller issues tend to be seen initially as an opportunity for learning, but if they continue or are numerous or serious enough they will be referred to a professional conduct committee. In general, the medical school will try hard to help you see where you went wrong and try and help you to ensure that things do not go wrong again.

If your professionalism is ever called into question, there are some ways that you can make the situation a lot worse. Firstly, not turning up to meetings that have been called to explore your professionalism does not go down well. Secondly, denial tends to suggest a lack of insight; 'it isn't cheating, everyone does it'. Finally, accusing the school of being pedantic or wasting time with professionalism rather than doing proper education is unwise: one student used the line 'don't you guys have anything better to do with your time than sitting around reading my Facebook comments?'

Assessment of professionalism by the GMC

Thankfully, we have no intention of summarising the GMC's plans for assessment of professionalism, as they are complex and likely to change in the near future. From a helicopter view, there seems to be the machinery for keeping things ticking over, monitoring for issues – these revolve around annual appraisal, cyclical revalidation, 360° appraisals and patient surveys; and then a different machine, the Medical Practitioners Tribunal Service (MTPS) that deals with those doctors who are suspected of having significant issues. The MTPS has a website listing details of recent decisions, which can be searched by keywords at www.mpts-uk.org/. It is worth looking through some cases, although it makes depressing reading. One recurring theme from the hearing reports is that the committee look very unfavourably on lying, lack of insight and lack of remorse.

There are cyclical calls to register medical students with the GMC, although at time of writing the professionalism of medical students remains under the remit of their medical school.

Acknowledgements

This chapter comes as a result of a multitude of discussions, arguments and debates with colleagues too numerous to name. However, particular thanks must be made to Bernadette John, the Digital Professionalism Lead at King's College, for sharing her up to the moment knowledge of digital professionalism and advice on cleaning up your digital footprint; Dr Julian Sheather, Deputy Head of Ethics at the British Medical Association, for running a thought provoking workshop on 'Social media – how not to get it wrong', that generated far more questions than answers; and to Dr Syed Naqi for his global perspective.

References and recommended reading

General Medical Council. (2009). *Medical Students: Professional Values and Fitness to Practise*. Manchester, GMC.

General Medical Council. (2013a). *Good Medical Practice*. London, General Medical Council.

General Medical Council. (2013b). *Maintaining a Professional Boundary between You and Your Patient*. London, GMC.

General Medical Council. (2013c). *Doctors' Use of Social Media*. London, GMC.

Medical Practitioners Tribunal Service, available at www.mpts-uk.org/ (accessed 24 February, 2015).

Royal College of General Practitioners (2013). *Social Media Highway Code*, London, RCGP

Other references

Evans, D. E. & Patel, N. G. (2012). *101 Things to do with Spare Moments on the Ward*. Oxford, Wiley-Blackwell.

Hilton, S. R. & Slotnick, H. B. (2005). Proto-professionalism: how professionalisation occurs across the continuum of medical education. *Medical Education, 39*(1), 58–65.

Justice Potter Stewart 'I know it when I see it': Jacobellis v Ohio, 378 US 184, 197 (U.S. Supreme Court 1964).

Chapter 13

Papadakis, M. A., Hodgson, C. S., Teherani, A. & Kohatsu, N. D. (2004). Unprofessional behavior in medical school is associated with subsequent disciplinary action by a state medical board. *Academic Medicine*, 79(3), 244–249.

Swick, H. M. (2000). Toward a normative definition of medical professionalism. *Academic Medicine*, 75(6), 612–616.

Wormald, B. W., Schoeman, S., Somasunderam, A. & Penn, M. (2009). Assessment drives learning: an unavoidable truth? *Anatomical Sciences Education 2*, 199–204.

Questions and answers

Q: I am part of a [social media] group for medical students, aimed at helping us learn. Some students discuss confidential patient data and even put pictures of patients up. No one seems bothered, should I do anything?

A: Yes. You must remind them about patient confidentiality and that online data is indelible. Regardless, they should try their hardest to delete any confidential data that they have posted; this may involve contacting the social media administration. There may be a group moderator or owner whom you can contact to express your concern. If they do not listen then leave the group and see if the professionalism lead in your medical school might want to take things further.

Q: In the operating theatres, the surgeon insists that all the students conduct a rectal or vaginal examination on the anaesthetised patient. It is good teaching, but I do not think the patient has given consent. I do not feel I can say 'no' to the surgeon, who is quite intimidating.

A: Vaginal or anal penetration of someone without consent when they are unconscious is a sexual assault, whether they are unconscious because of alcohol, drugs or anaesthetic. As well as being illegal, it destroys the fundamental relationship of trust that is so essential, particularly for a surgical patient (consider how you would feel if you were going to have a general anaesthetic). This situation is rare and thankfully becoming rarer; however, students can have difficulty in finding a strategy for saying no. Probably the easiest approach is to use the 'stuck record' response – say 'No, I'm sorry, I don't believe that the patient gave consent for me to examine them intimately, so I cannot do so' and keep repeating that phrase or variations of that phrase 'As I said, I'm really sorry, but because the patient didn't give consent, I cannot do so' until they give up. Go and see your professionalism lead, Dean of Students or equivalent as soon as possible. When considering the strength of persuasion that someone with power has over you, have a look online at the 'Milgram experiment'.

Q: I took a history and examined a patient in A&E, I have just seen that they have sent me a Facebook friend request. It's OK to say yes, isn't it? I have hundreds of friends.

A: This is fascinating and covered well in the RCGP Social Media Highway Code (p. 17, see *Recommended Reading*). Consider whether you would give the same patient your phone number (hopefully not) and now consider how much more information the patient can gain from your profile. The consensus seems to be to send a polite message thanking them for their friend request, but stating plainly that you are unable to accept it as it would breach your professional boundaries.

Q: Many years ago I put something very inappropriate on social media – what should I do?

A: Imagine that it is now 10 years time that it has resurfaced and caused you grief. Looking back what do you wish you had done? We guess the answer would probably be: try your hardest to remove it/have it removed and keep a record (for ever) of the steps that you took. Write a reflective piece on why you did it and how your views have changed, matured. Keep this and revisit it and add to it each year or so. Find someone in your medical school or university that you can talk to – perhaps a professionalism lead, ethicist or digital professionalism lead; disclose the details and ask for advice. Read about professionalism, aim to develop and demonstrate exemplary professionalism.

Chapter 14 **Thinking ahead: student-selected components, careers and electives**

OVERVIEW

This chapter provides an overview of some of the choices that you will need to make during your time at medical school that might affect your future career. There are some themes running through this chapter: these include consciously planning activities in order to inform your future career choices; being careful not to narrow your options too quickly and re-evaluating your career knowledge and career position often. As always, curiosity will serve you well; you will have a lot to learn from others, even if theirs is not your preferred career. The hardest message is that you should expect some disappointments along the way; things do not always turn out the way you expected on day one. Often, students' childhood dreams of being a psychiatrist, a paediatrician or whatever crumble to dust during clinical attachments in those specialities. Your aim, therefore, should not be to stick to one choice, but should be to make sure that things will turn out well and that your career is guided more by active choices and less by chance.

Careers in medicine

There are whole textbooks written about careers in medicine and whole departments of faculty employed to advise you. We are not intending to replace these valuable resources, indeed medical careers are currently very much in flux and are likely to remain that way for some time to come. The older systems of slowly advancing and then waiting around for the consultant

How to Succeed at Medical School: An Essential Guide to Learning, Second Edition.
Dason Evans and Jo Brown.
© 2015 John Wiley & Sons, Ltd. Published 2015 by John Wiley & Sons, Ltd.

or general practice partnership that you were going to keep for life are gone and in its place is a fast-track run-through system, which will probably result in specialists changing jobs far more often than previously.

These fast-track programmes require early decisions about careers: you will be expected in your foundation years to be making some decisions about where you want to end up 5 or 7 years later. This causes much stress to many. You can minimise this stress by being strategic at medical school and building a portfolio of experiences that will guide you to the areas that you are interested in pursuing and the areas that really do not 'do it' for you.

The current blurb for the fast-track systems is that there will be little flexibility; they will run like efficient conveyor belts, with FY2 doctors joining at the bottom and falling off the top as specialists. In reality, of course, humans are messy – they get sick, get pregnant, go off abroad for a year, emigrate halfway through their training or have even been known to *change their minds* halfway through training as to their preferred career. Any system will need to adapt to this messiness will need to become organic, even if this is not evident in the formal planning. In other words, there will *always* be second chances.

You should consider it as one of your main jobs at medical school, from day one, to be curious about other people's careers: ask every clinician you meet the story of how they reached their current position, ask them what the best bit and the worst bit of their job is. You might not want to do gynaecology for a career, but you can still learn a lot from the career path and choices that a gynaecologist made. When did they know that the career was for them? Did they take any career gaps? How did they know that they were ready to be a consultant? If you discover that everyone who you respect spent time abroad, for example, then you might feel more tempted to build that into your career plan as well.

> I don't know what kind of doctor I want to be. I'm really looking forward to the next few years and getting a real flavour of the range of options I have.
>
> Josh, first-year medical student.

Try and engage with all the medical specialities (including general practice, general medicine, general surgery etc.) that you are connected to as a student, and if you miss out on some, think of ways of finding out about them. One way is through arranging student-selected components (SSCs) as discussed in the next section, but there are other options too; talk to students who have been attached to those specialities, perhaps during some spare time you could hang around on their wards (introduce yourself to the nurses first) and see if you can shadow the junior doctors, ask to sit in on clinic or to go to the departmental meetings or training.

Some students feel awkward approaching clinicians to ask about careers. If this includes you, try the following exercise.

EXERCISE

Imagine that you are a specialist in one of the smaller specialities, let's say tropical neurology; you have spent your life pursuing this speciality, it is your vocation and your passion. Your one regret is that the medical school does not recognise its importance enough for it to be included on the medical student rotations. A medical student contacts you asking if he or she can meet with you to ask about tropical neurology as a career. How do you respond?

Student-selected components/modules

Thanks to the GMC (1993), almost every medical school curriculum in the United Kingdom comprises core material and optional components. These optional components, called different things in different institutions, commonly SSC or SSM (special study module), usually last for 2–4 continuous weeks, or alternatively may run a half-day or a day a week for 5 or 10 weeks. They are supposed to be opportunities to investigate a topic in more depth; you might, for example, have an SSC in embryology or haematology or sexual health. These SSCs will occur throughout your years at medical school, with some having a predominantly academic slant, others being more clinically focused. Within all this diversity, there are principally two types of SSC: formal ones and self-organised ones.

Off-the-shelf student-selected components

Most SSCs are offered as formal, school arranged, off-the-shelf affairs, where you read the description and put your name down. Usually there is some system of allocation that seems reasonably fair if you get your first choice and terribly unfair when you do not. When you look through the options, students commonly choose depending on interest, likelihood of getting their choice, ease of the course and suspected grade (SSCs where most students get the grade A seem remarkably popular). You might want to also add into this equation some thoughts about career. If you have always wanted to be a paediatrician since as early as you can remember, then perhaps an early SSC in paediatrics will be useful to see whether it is what you really expected. If you think that an academic career in research will be for you, then how about an SSC that involves some sort of research. Perhaps you will discover that you hate statistics or that academic writing is not for you. Better to find these things out early. If you cannot decide between obstetrics and gynaecology or pathology as a career, an SSC in each in your first couple of years will give you more information to help you decide.

Self-organised student-selected components

Self-organised SSCs can be particularly fruitful in helping you with career choices. The most important person here is the SSC officer/coordinator/administrator in the student office. This is someone to build a relationship with as they will know the regulations and the loopholes. Let us say that you are interested in paediatric surgery and yet there is no formal attachment or pre-existing SSC in that speciality; most medical schools will allow you to arrange your own, either at your home hospital or further abroad, so long as you follow certain rules. Get these in advance and piece together a proposal – you might want to send some e-mails off to paediatric surgery departments asking about the possibility of an attachment (make the e-mail enthusiastic but not too over the top), or you might want to talk to the SSC officer at your institution, he or she might know of other students who did a really good attachment with a certain surgeon:

Great students are those who are proactive. Many of the situations students face, whether they are academic or personal, can be resolved or managed, though are often left until they become unnecessarily difficult and complicated.

Students need to view approaching the Student Office as not a sign of their failure to achieve as an individual, but rather as taking a responsible and professional approach to managing their education, which in turn are both key qualities which should resonate throughout their future careers.

Mr Robert Sprott, Bart's and the London.

Cheek and charm are essential when arranging your own SSCs. This includes expressing your enthusiasm, commitment and good organisation when you are trying to arrange it, during it (sounds unnecessary to say, but you should attend 110% and engage with the team, the clinicians and the patients) and after. The period after the SSC is particularly important: write a brief, honest but constructive report and put it in your portfolio (Chapter 7). Send a copy (modified if necessary) to the person who supervised you, and consider keeping in touch with them, perhaps an e-mail every term updating them on your progress. They might be a useful contact in the future for references, summer jobs or careers advice. Importantly, also send a copy of

Chapter 14

the report to the SSC officer, thanking them for the help that they gave you in organising it (even if that help was not as great as it could have been). If you have arranged an SSC abroad, think about bringing back something local and inexpensive (Belgian chocolates if you were in Belgium, Swiss chocolates if in Switzerland, you get the idea) for the student office and let them know how it went. Next time you want to build your own SSC, the student office will know that you are the sort of student who will make the most of it and they are more likely to put themselves out to help.

When second best *is* good enough

It will happen more than once that you will be denied your first choice of SSC or even of clinical rotation. Rather than the paediatrics SSC that she was hoping for, student A finds herself 'trapped' in a General Practice SSC; ironically, student B is in the opposite situation. They tried to change, but realised that if they pushed it much further, they would fall out with the student office, so they decide to make the most of it. Some students in this situation will do the minimum necessary to pass the SSC and spend most of their time elsewhere, either in body or spirit. We would advise one of two other routes.

The first thing you could try is to throw yourself into this speciality, which was not your first choice. If you want to be a good hospital-based paediatrician, you will need to understand how general practice works pretty well – how else can you refer patients back for follow-up from their GP? In fact, it is hard to think of any speciality that does not require a clear understanding of other specialities. Indeed, things often fall apart when this is missing. So your first option is to throw yourself into the SSC and see what you can get out of it; you never know, you might even realise that you had some misconceptions about the subject and it is more interesting than you thought. Much as you might hate gastroenterology, you will see countless patients with bowel problems and need to explain endoscopy to hundreds of patients and probably a few simulated patients in exams, so an attachment in gastroenterology might be fruitful after all.

Your second option is to negotiate for a modification of the SSC. In our aforementioned example, where student A wanted a paediatrics attachment and got a GP attachment, she could ask to be involved with baby clinics, school visits, perhaps a young person's asthma clinic. Student B, who wanted an attachment in general practice but ended up with the paediatricians, could ask to do some community paediatrics clinics, outpatient clinics, perhaps do baby checks with the paediatric or obstetric senior house officer. Student A learns about paediatrics in general practice; student B learns some important skills for general practice within a paediatric attachment.

Remember, especially if people agree to bend the rules for you, to show that you are grateful for the opportunities that come your way.

Chapter 14

Electives

Tradition has it that medical students spend some time away, usually in their final year, to study in another institution for a prolonged period (variable between medical schools, but usually in the order of a couple of months). Most students choose somewhere exotic and combine study with travel and immersion in a different culture. Some students stay home, arranging attachments where they will be with a team long enough to take some responsibility and see practice in more depth than they ever had time to as a medical student.

Your school will provide support and guidance, and even some rules about arranging electives, and you should take full advantage of this, along with previous students' elective reports (usually to be found in the library, sometimes online or in the student office), and you will even find some books on electives abroad (see *Further Reading*).

Choosing an elective

Before choosing a country, or even a speciality, you might want to stop and think about what you want to get out of this period. Spend some time deciding on what the **goals** of the elective are. Be honest with yourself, you do not need to share this list of goals with anyone else, not before editing it. It might be that you are considering a career in nuclear medicine and you want to spend the time shadowing a nuclear medicine consultant to be sure that you know what they really do. Perhaps you are sure that you want to be an HIV physician and an opportunity to work in an HIV hospice in a developing country will help you recognise late complications of the disease, rarely seen now in the United Kingdom, and also will not do your job applications any harm. You may, however, have more personal goals in mind. Perhaps this will be your first time distant from home and for some it will be a chance to explore something about themselves as well as a different country; for others, it might be an opportunity to finally lay some demons from the past to rest, what better place to do this than trekking across the Himalayas.

Once you have set some goals, the possible locations become easier to choose. You will need to keep your options fairly broad so that you have multiple layers of suitable back-up plans, but be reassured that by this stage in your career you will be highly skilled at gathering information – just do not forget to talk to the others who might have been there before and look at some books as well as the Google searches!

Probably the most important thing for an elective is your supervisor. Finding the right supervisor, someone who is enthusiastic, will welcome you and provide guidance and mentoring, will make a major difference to your

Chapter 14

experience, regardless of whether you are in Guatemala or Southend-on-Sea. Speak to others who have worked with the same supervisor, look for recommendations and personal contacts of faculty (ask 'but what is he/she like as a person?' to get an indication) and see what sort of relationship you can build by e-mail.

Ethical considerations

If you are travelling far afield, you might need to pay particular attention to any ethical issues of your trip. If you are travelling to a medically under-resourced population, for example, and are likely to be given a great deal of autonomy and responsibility without support and supervision, then there are clear ethical issues. You might be able to find another institution in the same country where you will have better supervision. Similarly, if you are starting or getting involved with a project while abroad, perhaps providing healthcare or training, think about what will happen when you leave. It might be better not to start something that cannot be sustained.

There often are not clear rights and wrongs, but it is important that you consider the implications of your elective and that you talk this through with your peers and tutors. In years to come, this is a time to look back on with fond memories, not tinged with regret.

> I went on elective to a small hospital in Africa thinking that I would have a fantastic experience. It turned out that sometimes I was the only 'medical' person available, and I ended up having more responsibility than I could cope with. I'm not sure that it was the experience that I had hoped for.
>
> James, newly qualified doctor.

Funding

You might be surprised at the range of funding opportunities for electives. If you are performing a specific project, or if there is a significant level of personal development, funders are likely to be interested in supporting you. Speak to your student office about funding possibilities and even consider alternative sources such as industry, charities and professional bodies. This might be a good opportunity to learn how to write funding applications and remember, 'if you don't ask you won't get' – little harm in sending an enthusiastic letter or two out to potential funders.

Culture

Max Chevalier is an educationalist working with non-governmental organisations (NGOs) setting up rehabilitation training centres in post-conflict countries. As part of his unpublished master's thesis, he conducted a qualitative analysis of the experiences and perceptions of Dutch physiotherapists who travelled to developing countries on elective. Some students returned home enriched by the experience, valuing having been part of a different culture and gaining a huge amount of respect for health-care workers working in low resource settings, whereas other students returned with negative experiences, often with rather deep-seated prejudices that seemed to have developed while away. It was hard to find reliable predictors of a good outcome, but the following factors seemed helpful:

- having a good relationship with their supervisor or others who had worked or lived in the host country;
- having personal traits and approaches such as:
  - flexibility
  - a non-judgemental approach
  - empathy;
- knowing something about the country (including history and culture) before you go;
- knowing some of the local language;
- travelling in a pair: valued by many students, so that they had some safe 'space' in which to reflect on things that had happened, although some felt that this prevented them from engaging with local culture.

Aside from the supervisor, **curiosity** seems to be an important attribute for a positive outcome. Most students had a negative encounter of one sort or another – a supervisor shouting at them, for example. Those who, after enough time had passed for things to calm down, approached that supervisor and asked for help in understanding what they had done to cause offence, tended to have much better outcomes than those who withdrew. In Chapter 4, we discuss **feedback** in more depth, the same rules apply here: describe behaviours and try to avoid making premature judgements about meaning.

Michael Paige and colleagues (2006) have written a nice book, principally aimed at Americans studying abroad, which covers aspects of culture and cultural adaptation well. Your medical school library might have a copy of this or something similar. You can buy this book yourself directly from the University of Minnesota website.

Balance

Most students use the elective period to explore another country or culture and round the world tickets are popular. Do not forget that this is also an opportunity to explore a career in much more depth than you would usually

Chapter 14

be able to, and to explore the possibility of working in a different country; both of these opportunities are unlikely to ever be repeated, so make good use of them. Review your goals often, negotiate with your supervisor and make sure that they know where you are. If you have chosen your supervisor well, they will understand the need for you to take long weekends away from time to time.

Clearly, if you see your elective as just a holiday period, you will not only be losing out on a valuable experience but also run the risk of failing to reach an adequate assessment, which might lead to difficulties back home.

Follow-up

Consider keeping a diary or how about a blog? Many blogs allow you to e-mail or even text entries, which will make access easier if you are travelling or if Internet access is slow or intermittent. This will allow you to keep a record of events and reflections and might keep those at home reassured that things are going well.

Write up a report when you are on the way home, mentioning experiences good and bad, and add useful contacts' details. Think about what advice you would have found useful before going and write that in. You might want to include some personal reflections or you might prefer to keep them for yourself; it is still worth writing them down (see Chapter 7 on portfolios). Send thank-you letters to everyone and anyone involved, including a copy of the report. Some will read it, others will not, but it is likely that they will appreciate your thanks.

If stressful things have happened on the elective, think about discussing these with others – either your friends or more formally with your tutors. You might want to think how you will make it easy for your colleagues to talk to you, if they have had difficult experiences on elective.

Summary

We have tried in this chapter to suggest that, right from the start of your time at medical school, you consider a career angle on everything you do, without being career driven or being single-minded in your thinking. You will have a lot to learn from all your clinical attachments that will help your future career, regardless of what speciality you will follow, but only so long as you see each of these attachments as an opportunity.

References and further reading

General Medical Council. (1993). *Tomorrow's Doctors: Recommendations on Under Graduate Medical Education*. London, GMC.

Paige, R. M., Cohen, A. D., Kappler, B., Chi, J. C. & Lassegard, J. P. *et al.* (2006). *Maximizing Study Abroad: A Students' Guide to Strategies for Language and Culture Learning and Use.* Minneapolis, MO, Center for Advanced Research on Language Acquisition.

Questions and answers

Q: I was always certain that I wanted to be a psychiatrist, but I have just completed my fourth-year psychiatry attachment and I did not enjoy it at all. I have no idea what to do now.

A: This is a relatively common situation, students who join medical school with a certainty of a particular career path can have a real shock when they get to know that speciality in more depth and discover that it is not for them after all. Often, this rather drastically affects motivation and some students can get pretty depressed. These are normal reactions but they need to be followed relatively rapidly by a phase of re-evaluation. Think about going to see your careers advice service, talk to friends and spend time writing down the things you like in medicine and the specialities that you have tried that you enjoyed.

Q: It is coming up to finals and I still have not decided on a career – what do I do?

A: There are three sorts of students who find themselves in this situation. There are those who find it difficult to make a decision – they are 95% sure that they want to be a GP, but that 5% stops them from committing. Easy advice here, you just need to commit! Suck it and see. For students who cannot decide between two options (vascular surgery or plastic surgery), and have had attachments in both and asked around a lot, try and find a job that would provide a common entry point to either – such as a common 'general surgery' start to specialist training or even a teaching fellow or demonstrator job in anatomy, clinical skills and so forth. For those with absolutely no idea, then consider applying for a 'holding job' – perhaps a non-training post that will give you useful experience whatever you end up deciding on.

Q: What happens if I do not get the FY job that I wanted? Will my career be ruined?

A: No. There is a lot of stress between final-year medical students about gaining the most prestigious FY jobs. There is no harm in trying for these posts, but in years to come you are likely to look back and value posts where you had good supervision and training, where you learnt lots and had a positive experience. Strangely most 'prestigious jobs' do not tend to fit this description. The same works for job interviews: you will impress the panel more by describing what you did and what you learnt in a busy job rather than having done a professorial job where you learnt nothing.

Chapter 14

Index

How to Succeed at Medical School: An Essential Guide to Learning, Second Edition.
Dason Evans and Jo Brown.
© 2015 John Wiley & Sons, Ltd. Published 2015 by John Wiley & Sons, Ltd.